The Super Foods Diet

The Super Foods Diet

— Nature's most powerful foods for healing,
prevention and weight loss

ISBN: 1481870610
ISBN-13: 978-1481870610

Printed in the United States of America

The Super Foods Diet

*— Nature's most powerful foods for healing,
prevention and weight loss*

By Vic Shayne, PhD

*Edited by
Tasha Shayne*

"Dr. Vic Shayne's new book is a must-read for anyone interested in learning about natural health solutions that are as much based in scientific evidence as they are in the evidence of our senses. Who out there couldn't use a crash course in super foods that have been vetted for authenticity by one of the greatest nutrition experts of our time? In a marketplace overrun by exotic fad foods, with outlandish claims, it is refreshing and encouraging that some really do deliver as promised. Those, like myself, who have already developed great admiration for Dr. Shayne's penetrating perspective on nutrition, exemplified by his now classic book, Whole Nutrition, will greatly appreciate the way he has broken down the complex topic of healing and nourishing the body with these special foods into straightforward, actionable steps that we can easily incorporate into our everyday lives. I recommend this book as essential reading for anyone serious about taking back control of his/her health one bite at a time."

— Sayer Ji

Founder, GreenMedInfo.com,
the World's Largest, Open Access, Natural Medicine Database with
over 20,000 study abstracts indexed and growing daily.

Contents

Super Foods Are Super Cures

What ails you? We're living in a world where cancer, diabetes, obesity, arthritis, blindness, and flu epidemics are the norm rather than the exception. What's happening here? Researchers at all the major universities are scrambling to find causes and cures. But can we afford to wait for them to come down from the mountain?

The great news is that we don't have to wait. The answer to most health problems plaguing us today is right under our noses — and it's been here for thousands of years. The answer is Super Foods.

Super Foods have stood the test of time and have been examined, prodded, tested, and re-tested in the laboratories of prestigious institutions around the world. Scientists have found that these Super Foods hold the power to prevent and heal even our most disturbing diseases. And now the secret to health and longevity is no longer a mystery. You don't need drugs, vaccines, or any other scientifically created concoction in order to live life to the fullest and not be subject to the diseases and symptoms that are plaguing and killing everybody around you.

Super Foods are the answer. Both traditional and native usage, in addition to modern-scientific research, confirm their effectiveness.

Unlike most books you've ever read, you don't have to wade through all the pages to find out what to do. We're going to tell you right here and right now, in the beginning.

There are FIVE main things you need to do to avoid the diseases that even most doctors say cannot be cured:

1. Eat Super Foods on a daily basis.
2. Avoid human-made foods.
3. Maximize the purity of your environment.
4. Exercise a little bit every day.
5. Feed your spirit.

Is This Book for You?

The answer is yes! If you're looking to lose weight, gain weight, feel better, look better, recover from a disease, stop pain, or prevent illness, you'll be excited to know that there are Super Foods that will help.

Even if you buy into the idea that your illness is genetic, the five principles outlined above will change your life and health like nothing else. **Just remember: Drugs do not cure disease because NO health problems are caused by drug deficiencies**. Health problems are caused mainly by *nutrient* deficiencies, and nutrients come only from natural sources: food, air, soil, and water.

Super Foods Are Super Effective

In recent years, the term "Super Food" has been applied to a number of foods and herbs discovered to benefit the health in more ways than one, with scientifically proven effects. Super Foods are useful in preventing disease, providing energy, and combatting illnesses and symptoms. They possess great versatility in their actions. While researchers have done much to try to locate or pinpoint a specific ingredient within each Super Food, the consensus is that the power of these foods lies not in any one isolated chemical, but rather in the food, in its entirety. In other words, the nutritional benefits of Super Foods are not limited to their vitamins, bioflavonoids, minerals, or proteins. You have to have all of the nutrients intact to make them work at their best. It's like a clock—you have to have all the working parts to make it function, and if you remove any of the gears, you can't expect to know the time.

Many Super Foods end up being consumed in fads. This happens not only because health and diet companies advertise them like crazy, but also because universities and researchers are continually making discoveries about them that are publicized then exploited for profit. Unfortunately, far too often, whole foods end up undervalued, appreciated only for one or two isolated chemicals found within them. Think of those nutrients you hear about all the time, read on your cereal box, or see on pill bottles in the health section of your grocery store—resveratrol, vitamin C (ascorbic acid), beta-carotene, pyruvate, folic acid, whey protein isolate, CoQ10, creatine, nitrites, etc. These nutrients are *taken out of* whole Super Foods and sold separately as isolated chemicals. Why? Because chemicals are cheaper than whole foods and much easier to patent, control, standardize, and intensify than to sell as a complete unit. Just remember that there's no such thing as a resveratrol tree and that folic acid is not folate (folate is the natural nutrient in real food, but folic acid is a manmade creation). Further, taking a resveratrol pill is not the same as eating grapes or drinking red wine; just as eating folic acid-enriched cereal is not the same as eating a green, leafy vegetable. Whole foods are complex in their makeup, offering nutrients as part of a system for healing and protecting your body—a system that can't be dissected by scientists then duplicated using only a few (or none) of its original parts because ALL THE PARTS rely on one another to be totally effective.

11

Ancient Healing Meets Modern Science

Natural health care was the original form of treatment for all ailments thousands of years before modern medicine came into existence. Natural health care has been making a big comeback in the modern world. This isn't to say that today's medical science isn't valuable, helpful, or significant, but rather to note that there's much merit to a great deal of the practices that were used long before the invention of drugs, x-rays, surgery, lasers, CAT scans, vaccines, and injections. Ancient healing foods were used long before there were scientific means for proving what natural healers already knew by virtue of experience borne of observation.

For decades, the pursuit of balanced health has been usurped by careless lifestyles, junk-food diets, and live-only-for-today attitudes. Far too many people have come to lean on modern medical modalities to compensate for their offensive diets and lifestyles. People have divested themselves of responsibility for living and eating well and have placed responsibility on modern doctors to fix the results of their negligence. The decades between 1950 and 1980 were arguably the most offensive with regard to the advent of mass food processing, canned vegetables, powdered soups, artificial sweeteners, trans-fats, frozen foods, margarine spreads, and sedentary lifestyles.

The tide seems to be turning. Feeling the need to be proactive in directing the course of their health and healing, consumers are spending billions of dollars on organic foods, herbs, food supplements, and natural healthcare practitioners. People are realizing that they can play a role in disease prevention and eliminating much of the suffering that comes from neglecting one's health and eating a nutrient-poor, high-chemical diet.

Millions of people are now investing in their own health by exercising, avoiding toxins, consuming organic foods, caring for the environment (and thus helping to reduce pollutants), embracing good nutrition, and looking to modern medical science as a part of an overall health plan instead of a convenient crutch. Of course, not enough people have jumped on the bandwagon, as evidenced by the outrageous obesity and disease rate in the United States, but hopefully taking responsibility for one's health will continue to spread.

From the age of early humans, foods and herbs have been used to treat diseases, symptoms, and injuries resulting from accidents, a hostile environment, and warfare. True, some of the earliest approaches were based on superstitious and worthless treatments that hinged on a non-existent or poor understanding of how the body works. But a great number of these early practices did turn out to be reliable, even though the scientific method had yet to be developed to show why and how they worked. Now, in the twenty-first century, we are finally beginning to scientifically prove the validity of using foods, herbs, and other natural means to address illnesses and prevent disease. For example, sailors have known for centuries that lemons can cure scurvy; now—with the help of biochemistry, instrumentation, and testing—we know how this is possible. Scientific experimentation, research, and technology allow us to take a closer look at controlled environments in which nutrients and unseen molecules affect the body, kill cancer cells, protect against disease, bolster tissues, fight off free radicals, create cellular energy, transmit nerve impulses, and more. Thanks in great part to modern science, we can finally look into the past to recognize healing wisdom so we can then be confident in our natural healthcare choices. Furthermore, physicians are now able to incorporate natural health remedies and methods into their treatments, and practice integrative medicine—the best of both ancient and modern medicine worlds.

What Do Foods Have to Do with Health?

Nature, aided by the evolution of culture, ideas and techniques, and trial and error, offers the most logical, balanced, safe, time-tested, proven, and harmonious means of healing what ails us. Nature is amazing because, in a very large part, it holds the secrets to optimal health, disease prevention, and healthy cellular activity. Foods are what human bodies recognize as friendly substances. Drugs, on the other hand, are regarded by the human body as foreign invaders.

While natural healthcare has been resurrected to some degree, buyer beware. Following the rise in popularity of alternative healthcare, organic foods, and green living, a wave of big profit-driven-only corporations have jumped on the bandwagon and started confusing the issue, redefining the organic foods industry and stretching the truth by calling their own products "natural." They've also sunk a lot of effort into influencing government officials to forbid more ethical companies to advertise their ingredients as "wholesome," drug-free, and raw. Just one example of this involved a milk farmer who advertised on his packaging that his milk does not contain any hormones. Monsanto, the maker of artificial growth hormones for cows, took this statement to be a threat to its own drug-laden milk. The big company sued the little guy in a case that amounted to nothing less than, "You're making us look bad, and we're going to make you pay for the insult!!"[1]

It seems that where ethics are needed the most—in the food industry—they have been choked out by soulless profit-seekers. At the hands of dishonest, greedy corporations, modern science has railroaded the practice of nutrition to include many substances and techniques that are anything but natural. The word "nutrition" is flippantly thrown around by both modern doctors and (surprisingly) many "natural healthcare" practitioners who aim to practice it but fail to do so. Instead, these practitioners engage in pharmacology yet call it nutrition. They prescribe vitamin pills to squelch symptoms, ignoring the unique healing properties of nature's whole foods, herbs, sunshine, clean air,

---

[1] http://www.keepmainefree.org/monsanto.html

exercise, water, and relaxing silence. Why? Because there's big money in things you can control, patent, and stick in a box or a pill. The simple truth is that vitamin pills and amino acid powders are not natural in the same way that processed foods are not natural. If you want to see the confusion at work, merely pick up a supplement bottle—or even a loaf of bread—and study its ingredients. If you see the names of chemicals, you can be assured they're not foods, and that they're definitely not natural.

The natural healthcare movement is a financial threat to many corporations invested in artificial ingredients, processed foods, and chemical vitamins. So they like to argue that there is no science behind the healing power of foods. The argument is an old saw by now and is not valid. For the lazy and arrogant, there is no proof; for the open-minded and curious, there is plenty of proof. You should know, as evidenced in this book, that natural healthcare, as well as a wide array of curative foods and herbs, are indeed supported by sound, up-to-date science. Researchers are continuing to look into why (and how) so many of nature's herbs and foods heal, so they can lend credibility to age-old cures. In our high-tech era, researchers use leading-edge diagnostic methods to define the structure of illness and then measure the effectiveness of natural healing modalities. In more precise words, we can use modern science to figure out what's wrong and then use nature to correct the problem.

What We Don't Know Is A Lot
No doubt, sound science is a key consideration when you realize there are hundreds of books and web-based articles based on unproven, half-true, speculative, or suspect principles that run the gamut from muscle testing to crystals. Such things cannot be included in the genre of natural healing because they haven't even stood the test of time, let alone scientific validation.

There are many things that we still don't know or understand about how foods and nature heal, yet we do not necessarily want to discount what we've learned from tradition. Beyond nutrition and herbalism, researchers are only recently gaining insights into the healing power of light, energy, sound, meditative exercises, breathing, mental exercises, mind-body medicine, and other ancient modalities. What we don't know is a lot. Doctors need to admit this fact or they are not worthy of claiming that they are adherents of modern science.

What Do Foods Have To Do With Health?

"What do foods have to do with health?" Asking this question, whether rhetorically or literally, shows the disconnection our society has from anything that's actually natural. It also gives us a glimpse into why our society is facing such a decline in health, despite our amazing scientific prowess. Thanks to the effects of overpowering marketing efforts that have been promoting quick fixes, artificial ingredients, and foul-nutrition, the majority of Americans continue to live out of touch with nature, including the very nature of their minds and bodies, how they work, and what they need for optimal function.

Every cell of every organ in your body is affected by a combination of the foods you eat and by chemicals entering your body through your daily diet. Of course, you're also affected by whatever you put on your skin and thusly soak in from the environment (including acid rain; industrial runoff in rivers, gulfs, and oceans; and chemicals released from plastic bottles containing your beverages). It can be argued that you are also affected by light, colors, sounds, textures, temperature, climate, stress factors, interaction with others, age, physical fitness, attitude, altitude, and recreational activities. But make no mistake: your state of health is greatly affected by what you *fail* to eat that would give your cells the vital ingredients they need to heal and prevent illness.

It's obvious that we are complex beings living in a complex world. The best we can do is to optimize the factors over which we have control.

Reliability Of Natural Healthcare

Let's entertain for a moment that there are four main views about healthcare....

The first is "The Medical Paradigm" that favors drugs, injections, and surgery as the accepted means of treating symptoms and diseases. This avenue is really more aptly termed "medical *treatment*," as opposed to health*care*. Medical treatment involves an attempt to resolve health problems caused by poor nutrition, faulty lifestyle choices, the ingestion of toxins, and even iatrogenic illnesses (resulting from medical mistakes, drug side effects, etc.). Most often, medical doctors work to offset health conditions that could have been prevented with wisdom, effective ways of handling stress and emotional trauma, and healthful diets. In other words, doctors are preoccupied with treating problems that could have been avoided.

The second view of healthcare is what may be termed "The Wacky and Unsubstantiated World of Crazy Cures." Some people—perhaps as a backlash to modernity or impersonal modern medicine—too easily accept illogical, unproven, sometimes careless and dangerous methods for healing, diagnoses, and prescriptions. This "New Age" approach to healthcare isn't necessarily new at all. It can, in fact, contain modalities that have been around awhile but receives a great deal of negative attention in modern society—much of it rightly so, because this approach is the same kind of nonsense that harkens back to snake oil salesmen, blood-letting, and sorcery.

The third category is "Traditional Healthcare" and includes the use of native plants, herbs, poultices, and diets of indigenous cultures. There is much wisdom and experience in this category, even if science is still working to provide all the proof for why such modalities and substances work. Traditional healthcare also incorporates steam baths and sweat lodges, enemas, massage, breathing techniques, Tai Chi, yoga, and meditation—all of which have merit in concrete, physiological terms. Trial and error over centuries, and even millennia, has helped fine-tune these traditional healing practices.

Lastly, we have a middle, balanced healing ground between old and new. In this one, the lessons, experiences, and wisdom of native cultures for their tradition of healing meld with the great advances in

17

science, including diagnostics, emergency care, surgery, and a deep understanding of biochemistry, physiology, neurology, and so forth. This area that we call "Integrative Medicine" must extract itself from the close-minded, exclusive, and solely pharmaceutical-driven approach to treating diseases and symptoms. When we are able combine traditional medicine with scientific research and discovery, the end result is a form of healing, prevention, and lifestyle with some genuine merit, fewer side effects, more complete healing, and a holistic approach to health problems. The emphasis here is that the patients are regarded as more important than the institutions that treat them.

Traditional peoples have been using foods and herbs as medicine for thousands of years. But with the help of modern science, we can now see the value in these substances from a more enhanced perspective. We can better understand how they work on a deeper level that only a century ago was impossible to explain with certainty. With scientific instrumentation and clinical trials, we can separate the absurd from the plausible. And this is the greatest value of science's role in natural healing. Today there are doctors leading the way in light therapy, using advanced sensory equipment to study energy being emitted by cells, and showing how thoughts and emotions are processed by the brain and then manifested into physical illness. When we can marry the healing power of plants (as well as thought, relaxation, exercise, etc.) with the power of scientific methodologies, the offspring is a greater understanding of illness that can be addressed with natural solutions.

One more thing to consider as we look for scientific evidence to validate the use of foods as healing, preventive, and curative agents: Traditional usage and experience are as important as modern-day studies. Science is largely concerned with finding the same results when employing the same tests. Traditional medicine has done the same thing, showing that over the course of hundreds or thousands of years, certain plants have worked successfully enough for healing that these plants, when used in a consistent manner, will result in the same reliable effect. This is science being practiced in the "world laboratory," where the lab is the jungle, plains, and mountains, and the subjects are real people with obvious illnesses. On this basis of testing throughout generations with the same plants and measured dosages, we can see the value in traditional food and herb cures. Modern science is not the only means of declaring that such cures are effective and reliable, though too many medical doctors dismiss and defame them as nothing short of witchcraft or voodoo medicine. With each passing year, scientists are discovering the same results as their forebears and delving into the means and properties by which traditional plants heal.

On the other hand, for the sake of comparison, not so much can be said of some of the more dubious forms of healing borne of ignorance, hope, delusion, misguidance or magic. When a doctor tells you that he can diagnose you by testing the strength of your arm muscle, or when he recommends a newly discovered cure-all, there is no comparison to be made with the tried and true methodology of traditional medicine. To group both under the "alternative" umbrella certainly robs the traditional healing methods of their deserved respect. Too often, the media, consumers, and allopathic doctors confuse untested New Age practices with traditional medicine practiced by herbalists from a wide spectrum of indigenous cultures. We must be careful not to confuse, for example, the herbal wisdom or food cures from Traditional Chinese Medicine with, say, the unproven and relatively new practice of Reiki, in which a practitioner can become a "master" in less than a year. Does it make sense that a practitioner "combing your invisible aura" can affect the same benefits as taking a specific herb that's been proven effective for over two thousand years? Traditional Chinese Medicine may be strange to most westerners, but this does not obviate the fact that behind it are millennia of research, practice, record keeping, and consistent implementation of healing modalities.

Astrophysicist Carl Sagan, in his bestseller, *The Demon-Haunted World*, helps illustrate this point. He writes,

Quinine comes from an infusion of the bark of a particular tree from the Amazon rain forest. How did pre-modern people ever discover that a tea made from this tree, of all the plants in the forest, would relieve the symptoms of malaria? They must have tried every tree and every plant—roots, stems, bark, leaves—tried chewing on them, mashing them up, making an infusion. This constitutes a massive set of scientific experiments that moreover could not be duplicated today for reasons of medical ethics. Think of how many bark infusions from other trees must have been useless, or made the patient retch or even die. In such a case, the healer chalks these potential medicines off the list, and moves on to the next. The data of ethnopharmacology may not be systematically or even consciously acquired. By trial and error, though, and carefully remembering what worked, eventually they get there—using the molecular riches in the plant kingdom to accumulate a pharmacopoeia that works. Absolutely essential, life-saving information can be acquired from folk medicine and in no other way. We should be doing much more than we are to mine the treasures in such folk knowledge worldwide... Certain kinds of folk knowledge are valid and priceless.[2]

If you want to know whether a certain healthcare method or substance will work to alleviate your problem, you have to retain a certain degree of skepticism and ask important questions, such as where experiments and research have been performed and if the evidence gleaned from the scientific or traditional laboratory bears consistent results. Thousands of years of observation and testing of a food or herb cannot be compared with untrustworthy hearsay and vague rumors claiming that cancer can be cured with baking soda or made to disappear with a homemade energy machine. An AIDS test in a modern medical clinic cannot be supplanted by a diagnosis made by a muscle tester or psychic. And the juice from a tropical plant cannot be said to cure any known disease unless there is modern scientific proof or at least hundreds of years of successful traditional usage. History is a great teacher and science is a method of intelligent skepticism, so we need to require that new modalities and substances, whether natural or concocted, will stand up to tests that consistently challenge their reliability, safety, and effectiveness. If we don't, then we continue to be fooled over and over again at the risk of our health and happiness.

This is not to say that a new application cannot be found for an old food, but merely that in order to become reliable as a healing agent, some proof must be shown other than flimsy testimony that has not stood the test of time or the barrage of skepticism inherent in the scientific method. Further, although natural healthcare comes under the scrutiny of modern medicine and the media, we have to be fair when working for the common good. We have to be aware of iatrogenic illnesses (thousands of cases of side effects caused by medical treatment and drugs every year) as well as untested, potentially dangerous inventions, such as genetic engineering of foods that are pushed into widespread acceptance and application without adequate testing, fluoride in our water supplies (there is scientific testing that shows fluoride to be more dangerous than beneficial), pesticide

[2] Sagan, Carl, The Demon-Haunted World; Science as a Candle in the Dark, Ballantine Books, NY, 1996, p. 251-252

residues on our foods, and aspartame. Both natural healing and modern medicine must be put to the test and made to prove their safety and effectiveness.

Real Nutrition: A Complex Idea

There's a misunderstanding in our modern world that nutrition means vitamin and mineral pills. This is far from the truth. Nutrition refers to foods that nourish the health and provide sustenance. People have lived for thousands of years without vitamin supplements. Instead, what formed the basis of their healthcare was real, whole, pure food grown in natural conditions under the sun, in the soil, and in all kinds of weather. Foods are complex, containing many different nutrients and substances that the body has come to rely upon as friendly and helpful. On the other hand, vitamin pills are far from natural. There's no such thing as a vitamin bush, a niacin tree, an ascorbic acid flower, or a four-legged creature called a "retinol."

The global market value of vitamin pills, at the time of this writing, hovers at around 2.5 billion dollars a year, and is rising at an average annual growth rate of just under 1 percent.[3] What is this figure telling us? For one thing, it's a sign of people's involvement in their own healthcare—but it's also alarming when we contemplate the true definition of the word "nutrition" and realize that society is still missing the mark.

Mother Nature knows the difference—and certainly our bodies know the difference—between foods and everything else that's included under the umbrella of what has been loosely termed "nutrition." Vitamins in pills are not foods, hence, they are not nutrition; they are chemicals, not foods. Foods contain vitamins, but vitamins do not contain food factors (helper nutrients such as fiber, flavonoids, flavors, textures, trace mineral activators, etc.). Over the past couple of decades, there has been an explosion in vitamin usage. But we are not much healthier. What's wrong with this picture? People are popping vitamins, multivitamins, minerals, protein drinks, and parts of foods, but are still eating fast foods, artificial ingredients, too many meats and sugars, and far fewer nutrients than our distant ancestors. Since vitamins are not foods, and because people are eating nutrient-depleting and nutrient-deficient foods, people are still not getting the nutrition required by their cells. And when they get sick from this kind

---

[3] Food concepts help vitamin industry growth, Decision News Media, foodnavigator.com,16-Jul-2003

of lifestyle, they turn to prescription drugs, which still fail to give them the nutrition their bodies are calling for. Vitamins and drugs cannot replace foods because they are palliative and not nutritive.

Scientists cannot make food, although they are always tampering with it and trying to "enhance" it. Sure, scientists, in the grand tradition of author Mary Shelley's Dr. Frankenstein, try to duplicate food particles in their clean, white laboratories, but they fail miserably. No matter, however, people and practitioners alike continue to use vitamin and mineral pills because our modern society has been brainwashed into thinking that scientists surpassed Nature in wisdom, healing, and nutrition. Ridiculous! Arrogant? You bet! Your body knows the difference.

If we examine the nature of Nature, so to speak, we see just how absurd it is that some scientists and doctors are deluded into thinking that they can create substances better than what nature has to offer. Why? Because food nutrients are parts of living things, and living things cannot be created from chemicals in a laboratory. Nor can they be broken into pieces and still expected to function in the same way as the original, complex entity. Attempts to "improve" on living things usually results in unforeseen problems because mere human beings, no matter how brilliant or well-intentioned, lack the wisdom and ability to comprehend, duplicate and/or predict the complexity, variables, effects, shortcomings, mistakes, omissions, and ramifications of their creations. Nature developed her bounty through billions of years of evolution; scientists try to improve upon this by investing only a few years or so in a laboratory.

Nature's Foods Are Complex
Nature's foods are complex. "Complex" means involved or intricate, as in structure; complicated. This means that foods (and herbs) grown in nature contain substances that exist as part of a greater whole. These substances work together (synergistically) and are not found apart from one another. By analogy, a leaf is found on a plant, but never grows by itself; a feather is found attached to a bird, but it's not a living entity unto itself. We can say the same thing about food particles. Vitamins and minerals are found inside foods, but do not exist alone in nature. However, modern science, in all its self-proclaimed glory, funded and promoted by giant corporations, has fooled the populace into thinking that vitamins are natural, even though they are no longer contained within their original food "complex." This is crazy but true.

This begs another analogy. If you took apart a watch to see how it works, you would find all kinds of important parts, including springs, glass, pins and so forth. Each part works in harmony with each other part. None of these alone has any function once removed. Yet, when working together with the other parts, each plays an important role. If you smashed the watch apart with a polo mallet and had it analyzed, you would find that the broken pieces are chemically identical to those of the original, functioning watch. But any thinking human being understands that chemical makeup is not all that's needed to make the watch work. The watch has to be in one piece for all the little parts to work in harmony, to function. This is how vitamins, minerals and other food particles work: as a team. Unless still contained in their original complex within the food, vitamins do not function the same way, as intended by the wisdom, evolution, and harmony of nature and the human organism.

The issue of complexity is a cornerstone of natural health care and the practice of nutrition. If this is not made clear, then treating ourselves with unnatural, artificial chemicals, vitamins, drugs, and minerals starts to make sense, which it shouldn't. Dr. David Suzuki, author of several books and documentaries on ecology and the environment, writes, "Nature is a complex, interconnected system made up of countless (and as of yet many undescribed) parts."[4] These "undescribed parts," are obviously unknown by scientific definition, yet we know that some beneficial factors exist because of the changes they affect. As stated in a previous example, we knew that lemons cured scurvy long before we knew that lemons contained vitamin C. We've also just recently discovered that people eating the traditional Mediterranean diet are healthier than most others. Scientists have discovered that Mediterranean peoples' wine, grapes, sunny climate, and emotive lifestyles promote wellness. By analogy, we knew that dropping a rock off a cliff would make it fall straight down, thousands of years before Newton called this effect "gravity." We don't necessarily have to wait until scientists discover an active ingredient in order to realize that a particular food is beneficial. While science is an excellent tool for understanding and defining our universe and how it works, it is poor at inventing anything that surpasses that which is natural. And science more often than not falls short in explaining the

[4] Suzuki, David T., David Taylor, The Big Picture: Reflections on Science, Humanity, and a Quickly Changing Planet, p.73, Greystone Books, Canada, 2009

complex mysteries of life—in particular, the mysteries of the healing properties of nature's foods.

Much of what we know about the beneficial aspects of foods comes from traditional use—how certain foods across world cultures have been grown, harvested, and consumed for their health benefits. Of course, now that scientists have dissected foods biochemically, we have a greater understanding of the role of particular vitamins, minerals, amino acids, bioflavonoids, essential fatty acids, and other factors *within* foods that sustain life, protect against disease, and eradicate symptoms. But we still don't know everything, and scientists have failed in trying to duplicate, bypass, or surpass the wisdom of nature by creating artificial vitamin pills, drugs, and other chemical concoctions in an attempt to match nature's capacity for meeting our bodily needs. In the end, nature's innate "intelligence," balance, dynamism, and complexity, involving mysterious and unknown factors—all of which has evolved over millennia—is no match for the limited minds and instruments of man. And it's still better to eat an apple than swallow a bunch of isolated chemicals in pills for the sake of getting your proper nutrition.

Further, all human-made chemical concoctions, whether vitamin pills or drugs, always have side effects. This is because human beings, meaning scientists, cannot create or re-create living structures such as foods. Most attempts to "improve" upon foods have resulted in the creation of undesirable, and often unpredictable, negative chain reactions.

Simply put, food has been, is, and will continue to be your best medicine.

Less Confusion At The Food Store

It's been said many times (because it's true) that the best foods to eat are on the perimeter of the grocery store (fresh fruits and vegetables), while the least nutritious are located in the center aisles (processed, sugary, and frozen foods).

There are three main categories of produce offered in grocery stores:
1. **Conventional**: foods grown with modern farming methods that include the use of toxic chemicals, poisonous fertilizers, and even genetically engineered "Frankenfoods." Conventionally grown foods can (and do) make people sick. Further, they are used as ingredients in the manufacture of processed foods, which, as far as our bodies are concerned, aren't really foods because they are overcooked, fortified with artificial vitamins, and made to sit on a shelf for months to years without rotting. When you buy conventional foods, you can't be certain of the food's quality because making a profit is more important to the manufacturer than protecting your health.
2. **Organic**: foods that are grown without toxic pesticides or fertilizers. Not too long ago (perhaps as recently as fifteen years in the past), the majority of organic foods were grown by people who care about the environment. They wanted a clean, pure, and nontoxic way of eating, not only to improve and nourish the health of people and animals, but also the earth, keeping artificial chemicals out of the human body and out of the soils and waterways. Now the organics industry is heavily tainted, so you have to do a little homework to protect yourself. Since big conventional food companies discovered that millions of people are interested in organics, they wanted in on the profit-making. So, what did they do? They started buying up small organic companies like Celestial Seasonings, Horizon, Cascadian Farms, and so forth. Unfortunately, too many people in big companies have small minds and cannot really understand or appreciate the importance of keeping chemicals away from people, animals, and the environment. Bottom line: They cheat for the sake of profits. Over the past two decades,

26

they've purchased most of the big organic companies and have since been working to bend the rules, change laws, change the meanings of labels, and lie about their ingredients and their standards. Can you trust organics anymore? Not unless you do a little research and familiarize yourself with which companies have sold out and which companies still have integrity.

3. **Biodynamics**: this is your best bet when it comes to wholesome, clean food. According to Organic Consumers Association (OCA) (which, at the time of this writing, is an association promoting organic and biodynamic farming, and the health of our planet), "We gain our physical strength from the process of breaking down the food we eat. The more vital our food, the more it stimulates our own activity. Thus, Biodynamic farmers and gardeners aim for quality, and not only quantity."[5]

The Organic Consumers Association reports:

"Chemical agriculture has developed short-cuts to quantity by adding soluble minerals to the soil. The plants take these up via water, thus by-passing their natural ability to seek from the soil what is needed for health, vitality and growth. The result is a deadened soil and artificially stimulated growth. Naturally occurring plant and animal materials are combined in specific recipes in certain seasons of the year and then placed in compost piles. These preparations bear concentrated forces within them and are used to organize the chaotic elements within the compost piles. When the process is complete, the resulting preparations are medicines for the Earth which draw new life forces from the cosmos...Two of the preparations are used directly in the field, one on the earth before planting, to stimulate soil life, and one on the leaves of growing plants to enhance their capacity to receive the light. Effects of the preparations have been verified scientifically."[6]

---

[5] What is Biodynamics? Based on An Introduction to Biodynamic Agriculture, originally published in Stella Natura 1995, Organic Consumers Association, organicconsumers.org, 2013

[6] Biodynamic Food & Farming, What is Biodynamics? Organic Consumers Association, 2008

Biodynamic Is Good For The Earth, As Well As The Consumer:

> "In his Agriculture course, Rudolf Steiner [father of biodynamic farming] posed the ideal of the self-contained farm - that there should be just the right number of animals to provide manure for fertility, and these animals should, in turn, be fed from the farm. We can seek the essential gesture of such a farm also under other circumstances. It has to do with the preservation and recycling of the life-forces with which we are working. Vegetable waste, manure, leaves, food scraps, all contain precious vitality which can be held and put to use for building up the soil if they are handled wisely. Thus, composting is a key activity in Biodynamic work. The farm is also a teacher, and provides the educational opportunity to imitate nature's wise self-sufficiency within a limited area. Some have also successfully created farms through the association of several parcels of non-contiguous land."[7]

The conclusion? Eat organically and/or biodynamically (preferable) grown foods from trusted growers to avoid disease-causing chemicals and ensure a greater degree of nutritional content in your foods. And don't eat artificial ingredients, refined sugars, food colorings and dyes, preservatives, artificial sweeteners, and trans-fats. Your body is a natural entity, so it needs natural foods to survive in health.

---

[7] ibid

Bite Into a Rainbow for Better Health

A number of old time nutritionists such as Bernard Jensen, Euel Gibbons, and Henry Bieler, MD, have written about the need for people to eat an array of colorful fruits and vegetables. Why would colors matter? What's the difference, you may wonder, between a green zucchini and a yellow squash? Orange carrots or blue berries? All the colorful foods you can think of, in their vast variety, have one main thing in common: value in their pigmentation. Colors matter.

Consider These Colorful Food Notes:
Natural pigments that give certain fruits and vegetables a rich red, purple, orange, yellow, golden, green, or blue color are potent anti-cancer agents. Ohio State University researchers discovered that compounds in foods such as eggplants, red cabbage, elderberries, and bilberries restrict the growth of cancer cells and, in some cases, kill them off entirely, leaving healthy cells unharmed. Researchers said foods with the highest levels of such compounds were most effective at slowing cancer growth, with exotic purple corn and chokeberries stopping the growth of colon cancer cells and killing 20 percent of the cells in lab tests. Radishes and black carrots slowed the growth of colon cancer cells by up to 80 percent.[8] Such findings bring scientists closer to unraveling the key ingredients responsible for giving fruit and vegetables their cancer-fighting properties. Because the pigments, representatives of the class of antioxidant compounds known as anthocyanins, are not easily absorbed by the bloodstream, they travel through the stomach to the gastrointestinal tract, where they are taken up by surrounding tissues to promote healing and fight disease.[9] In laymen's terms, after eating them, these antioxidants go right to the place in your body where they are needed the most.

---

[8] Wagner, Holly, "COMPOUNDS THAT COLOR FRUITS AND VEGGIES MAY PROTECT AGAINST COLON CANCER," The Ohio State University, COLUMBUS, Ohio, Aug 2007
[9] Sample, Ian, "Food pigments stop cancer in its tracts," *Sydney Morning Herald*, Aug 07

Tomatoes contain lycopene, one of a family of food pigments called carotenoids that occur naturally in fruits and vegetables. Lycopene gives tomatoes, watermelons, and pink grapefruits their red coloring. Antioxidants are a group of vitamins, minerals, and plant substances that play a key role in protecting our bodies from serious illness, particularly heart disease and cancer. Once absorbed into the body, lycopene helps prevent and repair cell damage caused by free-radical formation and oxidation.[10]

Carotene is an orange pigment needed in plant photosynthesis and protects your eyes, lungs, blood vessels, and skin, as well as against cancer. Your main dietary sources include orange and yellow fruits and vegetables, such as (as the name suggests) carrots, sweet potatoes, mangos, and cantaloupe. Carotenes are also in green, leafy vegetables like spinach, kale, and chard.

Beta-carotene is the most abundant and best known of all the carotenes and almost always occurs in nature accompanied by its lesser-known carotene siblings: alpha, gamma, delta, and epsilon. In nature, carotenes are also often found alongside other natural food pigments, such as xanthophylls, anthocynanins, and chlorophyll.[11]

The chlorophyll-rich carbohydrate parts of green vegetables create an environment inside our bodies that's hostile to the growth of fungi and mold. Chlorophyllin, a derivative of chlorophyll, is the green-colored element that enables plants to grow. It is the green you see in green vegetables, green tea, and many other green plants that possess preventive and medicinal value. George Bailey, PhD, Biomedical Sciences Center, Oregon State University, and his team of researchers found that chlorophyllin reduces the incidences of liver cancer in trout. And, when studying a population in China that had an unusually high incidence rate of liver cancer, they found that chlorophyllin, when added to the population's diet, reduced incidences of liver cancer by 50 percent. Chlorophyllin also reduces the body's absorption of aflatoxins (poisons caused by molds in foods) and eliminates them.[12]

Among the many pigmented foods that work to bolster your health are green tea, radishes, wild pansies, dandelions, beets, squash,

[10] "You Say Tomato, I Say Healthy," Thunder Bay Regional Health Sciences Centre, Canada
[11] Moss Report, Jul 08
[12] Fox, Maggie, Obese Americans now outweigh the merely overweight, Reuters, reuters.com, Jan 9 09

spinach, turmeric, cumin, berries, and even red wines. The most important concept here is that the colors in natural foods are representative of the nutrients found within them that fight and prevent cancer and diseases of the heart, liver, eyes, lungs, colon, skin, pancreas, and so forth. Powerful antioxidants in pigmented fruits, vegetables, seeds, nuts, and berries, as well as in fish such as salmon, all work to protect your cells from oxidative damage.

Super Foods Help You Lose Weight

Americans are spending billions of dollars every year to find out how they can lose weight. That's a lot of money. But, ironically, even with all this obsessing over *how* to lose weight, the United States is still an obese country. *USA Today* reports that 20 percent of preschoolers are obese. That's one-in-five children who are only four years old. MSNBC reports that the number of obese American adults is greater than the number of those who are merely overweight. Figures posted by the National Center for Health Statistics show that more than 34 percent of Americans are obese, compared to 32.7 percent who are overweight. Less than 6 percent are "extremely" obese. More than one-third of adults—72 million people—were obese in 2005-2006.[13]

Researchers at the University of California–San Diego School of Medicine and San Diego State University say that a lack of physical activity was the most significant risk factor contributing to obesity in eleven– to fifteen-year-olds. Interpretation: Kids are sitting on their butts watching TV and playing video games instead of engaging in sports and running around the yard or the park.

How can it be that we as a nation are so diet-conscious, while at the same time so miserably overweight? The answer may lie somewhere between these facts:

- People gain weight, then lose it, and then gain it again, so they become lifetime customers of the swelling (pardon the pun) weight-loss industry.
- The obesity rate continues to grow, creating an ever-new source of weight loss industry business and customer base.
- People are more weight-conscious than they are health-conscious; it's become an image thing and not a health issue.
- It's easier (so it seems) to cycle in and out of weight loss than to actually stay on a steady, healthy course.
- People are addicted to unhealthy foods.
- People are becoming less and less physically active.

---

[13] ibid

- Our country's federal government allows the makers of bad, sickening foods to advertise as if they are offering foods worth eating

Remember these five facts and you'll be on your way to losing weight the healthful way:

1. Eat fewer calories (if you eat less, you'll burn more).
2. Exercise daily. Engage in an activity that raises your heartbeat and respiration.
3. Eat fewer carbohydrates (unused carbohydrates are stored as sugar and fat).
4. Think about health first, weight second.
5. Detoxify your body with exercise and the foods you eat (foods with toxins are stored in fat cells; when your body holds onto the toxins, it also holds onto fat). When you eat Super Foods, your body eliminates toxins and therefore loses weight.

Antibiotic Super Foods

Prescription antibiotics are used and, in fact, overused for a great array of illnesses ranging from respiratory infections to the common cold. You may have read that antibiotic drugs can take their toll on your gut. This is due to their destruction of good bacteria which are essential to digestion and immune system health. When antibiotics kill off good bacteria, the result is often an overgrowth of yeast (called *Candida albicans*), which can lead to a lot of problems, including a lowered immune system, yeast infections, jock itch, thrush, athlete's foot, rashes, allergic reactions, frequent colds, digestive difficulties, and much more.

Antibiotics are often prescribed indiscriminately by physicians, leading to their misuse. Antibiotic drugs are often prescribed in cases of viral diseases, which is senseless because they have no power against viruses (they are anti-bacterial, not anti-viral).

Few people are aware that you don't even have to take prescription drugs to consume antibiotics. If you're looking to avoid antibiotics, you should know that non-organic beef, chicken, turkey, and other meats (including farm raised fish) contain varying levels of these drugs.

Even when antibiotics may be helpful at times to overcome health concerns, there are drug-free sources in Super Foods that are less destructive. A number of natural foods and herbs contain natural antibiotic and anti-fungal properties. In fact, there are a lot of them.

IMPORTANT SAFETY NOTE: Some herbs are very potent and may cause side effects—including compromising liver health—so it's always important to conduct a lot of research to make sure you're not causing more harm than good by taking one. It's always advisable to work with a qualified, experienced practitioner when using herbs.

Here Are A Few Anti-Microbial Super Foods And Herbs:

- Garlic[14] [15]
- Olive leaf extract[16]
- Turmeric
- Cilantro
- Australian tea tree oil
- Coconut oil (also called "coconut butter")
- Oregano oil Astragalus[17]
- Pau d'arco
- Cat's Claw
- Bentonite clay (this is not a food, but a natural clay)
- Honey (don't use it with yeast problems because of its sugar content)
- Noni[18]
- Neem
- Aloe vera

Rainforest Herbs:

- Picao preto
- Mullaca
- Anamu
- Brazilian peppertree
- Fedegoso

Rainforest Herbs That Specifically Target Yeast:

- Anamu
- Avenca
- Brazilian peppertree

---

[14] Gowsala P. Sivam, Journal of Nutrition, Protection against Helicobacter pylori and Other Bacterial Infections by Garlic, Bastyr University, Research Institute, Kenmore, WA

[15] Journal of Applied Microbiology, Volume 84 Issue 2, Pages 213 - 215; Sensitivity of food pathogens to garlic (Allium sativum)

[16] Balch, Phyllis, Olive Leaf, Prescription for Herbal Healing, p 103

[17] University of Maryland Medical Center, "Astragalus," umm.edu/altmed/articles/astragalus-000223.htm

[18] United Nations Foundation, Plant Component Kills Bacteria, Researchers Say, December 21, 2000

- Clavillia
- Guaco
- Guava
- Jatoba
- Mulateiro
- Pau d'arco
- Picao preto
- Stevia

There are many more foods and herbs that offer anti-bacterial benefits. Good sources for locating them can be found listed in Dr. James Duke's books, including his bestseller, Green Pharmacy.

Why Begin With Broccoli?

Whenever nutritionists talk about the best foods for the body, it seems as though they typically begin with broccoli. Well, there's no getting around the fact that broccoli is a leader in the Super Foods category. There are broccoli florets (the flowery parts of the vegetable that are most commonly eaten by broccoli eaters), broccoli sprouts (the broccoli plant that's just peeking out of the ground), and broccoli sprout extracts. All of these offer a super array of healing and protective features. At the top of the list is broccoli's power to prevent cancer.

"Cancer is a health problem of enormous global magnitude," said Dr. Paul Talalay of Johns Hopkins University School of Medicine. "It has been very difficult to demonstrate substantial clinical progress in the last 25 years, despite spectacular advances in our understanding of the causes, the nature and the molecular pathology of the disease." Talalay said that diet-focused strategies to protect against cancer and combat its development are showing significant promise. The value of cruciferous vegetables, like broccoli, are among the most notable cancer-fighters, and recent studies have also found that very young broccoli sprouts may have even greater value because they contain a stronger concentration of nutrients.[19]

During the American Association for Cancer Research's 4th annual *Frontiers in Cancer Prevention Research* meeting in Baltimore, Maryland, five studies were presented and added to the arsenal of research showing that the inclusion of certain vegetables and herbs in the diet can prevent or, in some cases, halt the growth of cancer. What's significant is that this is not just a matter of mechanical prevention, such as adding fiber to the diet to maintain digestive health and help you eliminate wastes. The research for these studies involves the chemical interactions between compounds found in foods, such as broccoli and other cruciferous vegetables (cabbage, cauliflower, kale,

---

[19] OSU News, Oregon State University, Corvalis, OR, oregonstate.edu/dept/ncs/newsarch/1999/Apr99/cancer.htm, Ap 12 99

etc.), and the body's cells and DNA. Clearly, adding these powerful foods to the diet can reap benefits at any stage of life.[20]

Oregon State University's Linus Pauling Institute found sulforaphane—a compound found in cruciferous vegetables such as broccoli, bok choy, and Brussels sprouts—contains strong anti-cancer properties. Even more promising results have been found in broccoli sprouts. These tiny, thread-like sprouts, sold in many stores alongside alfalfa sprouts and bean sprouts, have more than fifty times the amount of sulforaphane found in mature broccoli.[21]

Scientists at the University of California–Santa Barbara (UCSB)—laboratories of Leslie Wilson, professor of biochemistry and pharmacology, and Mary Ann Jordan, adjunct professor in the Department of Molecular, Cellular, and Developmental Biology—have shown how the healing power of these vegetables works at the cellular level:

> Breast cancer, the second leading cause of cancer deaths in women, can be protected against by eating cruciferous vegetables such as cabbage and near relatives of cabbage such as broccoli and cauliflower," said author Olga Azarenko, a graduate student at UCSB. "These vegetables contain compounds called *isothiocyanates*, which we believe to be responsible for the cancer-preventive and anti-carcinogenic activities in these vegetables. Broccoli and broccoli sprouts have the highest amount of the isothiocyanates. Our paper focuses on the anti-cancer activity of one of these compounds, called sulforaphane, or SFN," Azarenko added. "It has already been shown to reduce the incidence and rate of chemically induced mammary tumors in animals. It inhibits the growth of cultured human breast cancer cells, leading to cell death.[22]

Steven Clinton, associate professor of Hematology and Oncology, Ohio State University, said, "There's no reason to believe that this is the only compound in broccoli that has an anti-cancer effect.

---

[20] Tait, Elizabeth, Broccoli Sprouts, Cabbage, Ginkgo Biloba and Garlic: A Grocery List for Cancer Prevention, American Association for Cancer Research, Baltimore, MD, aarc.org, Oct 31 05

[21] Oregon State University, Eat Your Broccoli: Study Finds Strong Anti-Cancer Properties in Cruciferous Veggies, Corvallis, OR, May 5, 07

[22] Gallessich, Gail, Scientists Show Certain Vegetables — Like Broccoli — Can Combat Cancer, 93106, University of California, Santa Barbara, Vol 19, No 8, Jan 12 09

There are at least a dozen interesting compounds in the vegetable. We're now studying more of those compounds to determine if they work together or independently, and what kind of effects they have on cancer cells."[23] Clinton and his colleagues have been building upon the work of researchers from Harvard to show broccoli's effects against bladder cancer, who discovered that men who ate two or more half-cup servings of broccoli per week had a 44 percent lower incidence of bladder cancer when compared to men who ate less than one serving each week.[24]

Broccoli has also shown promise for prostate cancer because it contains substances acting as a powerful anti-androgen, inhibiting the rapid growth of human prostate cancer cells. Androgens comprise a class of male hormones that are important for the normal development and function of the prostate, but they also play a villainous role in the early stages of prostate cancer, and are typically treated with anti-androgen drugs. In most cases of prostate cancer, cancer cells develop resistance to androgen and grow independently of the hormone in later stages of the disease. University of California–Berkeley scientist Hiel Le said the incidence of prostate cancer among men in Asia—where consumption of vegetables is higher—is significantly lower than that for men in the United States. However, the risk for male Asian immigrants rises to levels comparable to American men the longer they stay in the United States, suggesting that factors such as diet and lifestyle play a role in the development of prostate cancer. "There are already plenty of health reasons for consuming more vegetables such as broccoli," said Le. "This study suggests that there are even more benefits to a diet rich in these phytochemicals when it comes to preventing prostate cancer."[25]

Research published in the *Journal Clinical Immunology*, shows that broccoli's sulforaphane triggers an increase in the amount of antioxidant enzymes released into the human airway (pathways to the lungs), which, in turn, offer protection against the onslaught of free radicals breathed in everyday from air pollution, pollen, diesel exhaust, and tobacco smoke. As a supercharged form of oxygen, free radicals can cause oxidative tissue damage, leading to inflammation and

---

[23] Schwartz, Steven, Broccoli Packs Powerful Punch to Bladder Cancer Cells, Ohio State University Research News, COLUMBUS , Ohio, 2009
[24] ibid
[25] Yang, Sarah, Chemical in Broccoli Blocks Growth of Prostate Cancer Cells, New Study Shows, UC Berkeley News, 12 May 03

respiratory conditions like asthma.[26] That's bad. But the good thing is that broccoli is nature's super hero.

"We found a two- to three-fold increase in antioxidant enzymes in the nasal airway cells of study participants who had eaten a preparation of broccoli sprouts," said Dr. Marc Riedl, David Geffen School of Medicine at UCLA. "This strategy may offer protection against inflammatory processes and could lead to potential treatments for a variety of respiratory conditions."[27]

Broccoli is highly valuable—not only as for your respiratory system, but also for supporting detoxification, and as a supply of vitamin K (and other vitamins) and sulfur (among other minerals).

---

[26] "Broccoli May Help Protect Against Respiratory Conditions Like Asthma" ScienceDaily (Mar. 4, 2009)

[27] Liu, PhD, David, "Broccoli compound may help prevent respiratory inflammation," foodconsumer.org, Mar 2, 2009

Tomatoes Protect Blood Vessels

Lycopene is a bright red carotenoid pigment and phytochemical found in red fruits and vegetables such as red carrots, watermelons, papayas, and most notably, tomatoes (but not strawberries or cherries). It keeps your blood vessels pliable, preventing cardiovascular disease, bypass surgeries, heart attacks, plaque build-up, and poor circulation.

According to a study published in the medical journal *Atherosclerosis,*[28] women with the highest levels of lycopene also had lower LDL (low density lipoprotein) cholesterol ratings. LDL is used by the medical industry as an indicator of heart disease. Lycopene helps LDL resist destruction by oxidation[29] and, as noted by researcher Jong Ho Lee from the Department of Food and Nutrition at Yonsei University, South Korea, it prevents atherosclerosis (damage to blood vessels), which in turn is believed to prevent stroke and heart disease.[30]

Unlike other fruits and vegetables, where heating tends to lower certain nutritional content, such as vitamin C, cooking tomatoes actually increases the amount of lycopene available to be used by your cells. Lycopene in tomato paste is four times more bioavailable (useful) than in fresh tomatoes. Tomato products such as tomato juice, soup, sauce, and ketchup contain the highest concentrations of bioavailable lycopene of all tomato-based sources.

Eating tomatoes that have been cooked and crushed (as is done in the canning process) or used in oil-rich dishes (such as spaghetti

---

[28] Daniells, Stephen, "Lycopene linked to healthier blood vessels," NutraIngredients newsletter, Aug 09, citing *Atherosclerosis*, published 13 August 2009, doi: 10.1016/j.atherosclerosis.2009.08.009, "Independent inverse relationship between serum lycopene concentration and arterial stiffness", Authors: H.Y. Yoe, O.Y. Kim, H.J. Kim, J.K. Paik, J.Y. Park, J.Y. Kim, S.-H. Lee, J.H. Lee, K.P. Lee, Y. Jang, J.H. Lee

[29] Oxidation is a term that is used quite commonly regarding disease causation, and is familiar to chemistry. When certain molecules (such as molecules of poisonous substances in the cells or bloodstream) come into contact with others, they can steal their oxygen. The reaction to this event may result in the production of free radicals, which start chain reactions that damage cells. Antioxidants put a stop to these chain reactions and thereby fight disease, support cellular structures and bolster the immune system.

[30] ibid

sauce or pizza) greatly increases the body's ability to pull this carotenoid from the digestive tract into the bloodstream, where your body finds the most use for it. Lycopene is fat-soluble, so the oil from other foods cooked along with the tomatoes can help its absorption.

Berry Good for Your Health

It has long been established that fruits and vegetables should make up the bulk of the diet. But the role of berries has been overlooked until very recently because berries aren't always categorized as fruits, and they're certainly not vegetables. More and more evidence continues to mount in favor of adding berries to the diet as a way of greatly enhancing your health and potentially warding off disease.

Within the last decade or so, scientists have shown that berries can offset the free radicals (oxygen robbers) that damage blood vessels needed to feed the heart, eyes, and extremities. Thus, as one example of berry power, bilberries have been studied and noted to prevent debilitating eye diseases. Free radicals come from toxins, heavy metals, and other sources and can erode tissues, cause cancer, and foment disease.

Berries are antioxidant foods and should be part of a good diet, as they are credited with preventing coronary artery disease, some cancers, macular degeneration, Alzheimer's disease, and some arthritis-related conditions.

Cancer is one of the greatest areas of berry research, since berries seem to show much promise in causing the death of cancer cells.

"Strawberries may be the most effective of the five most commonly consumed berries at inducing cancer cell death," according to a recent study conducted at the UCLA Center for Human Nutrition. "The center recently tested extracts of six berries—strawberries, raspberries, black raspberries, blueberries, blackberries and cranberries—to determine their ability to induce apoptosis, a process that enhances the death of cancer cells....Strawberries and other berries contain high levels of the phytochemicals that are believed to be responsible for the protective effects of diets high in fruits and vegetables against chronic illnesses such as cancer, inflammation, heart disease, and neurodegenerative diseases."[31]

---

[31] "Strawberries most effective at inducing cancer cell death," news-medical.net, Aug 05

The *Journal of Agricultural and Food Chemistry* reports, "Research suggests that the *polyphenolic* compounds found in berry fruits, such as blueberries and strawberries, may exert their beneficial effects either through their ability to lower oxidative stress and inflammation or directly by altering the signaling involved in neuronal [nerve] communication, calcium buffering ability, neuroprotective stress shock proteins, plasticity, and stress signaling pathways. These interventions, in turn, may exert protection against age-related deficits in cognitive and motor function."[32] In short, berries protect nerves, help cells communicate with one another and support mental functions.

How Many Berries Can You Name?

An overwhelming body of research firmly establishes that the dietary intake of berries has a positive and profound impact on human health, performance, and disease. And, as luck would have it, the number of berry types is astounding! Berries, which are commercially cultivated and commonly consumed in fresh and processed forms in North America, include blackberries, black raspberries, blueberries, cranberries (i.e., the American cranberry, Vaccinium macrocarpon, distinct from the European cranberry, V. oxycoccus), red raspberries, and strawberries. Other berry fruits, which are lesser known but consumed in the traditional diets of North American tribal communities, include chokecherries, highbush cranberries, serviceberries, and silver buffaloberries. In addition, berry fruits such as arctic brambles, bilberries (also known as bog whortleberries), black currants, boysenberries, cloudberries, crowberries, elderberries, gooseberries, lingonberries, loganberries, marionberries, Rowan berries, and sea buckthorns, are also popularly consumed in other parts of the world. Recently, there has also been a surge in the consumption of exotic "berry-type" fruits such as pomegranates, goji berries (also known as wolfberry), mangosteens, Brazilian açaí berries, and Chilean maqui berries.[33]

---

[32] *J. Agric. Food Chem.*, 56 (3), 636–641, 2008. 10.1021/jf072505f
[33] *J. Agric. Food Chem.*, 56 (3), 627–629, 2008. 10.1021/jf071988k

The Remarkable Bilberry

Bilberries are the European versions of blueberries. In fact, they look the same as blueberries and have been used traditionally in flavorful desserts and nutritiosaidnal medicines alike. This special berry is a healthful antioxidant,[34] offering the benefits of other vitamin C foods to protect smooth tissues, blood vessels, and the eyes. Herbalist James Duke, PhD, said that bilberry is a vasodilator responsible for widening the space inside blood vessels and lowering blood pressure.[35]

Researchers at the University of Maryland Medical Center write, "Bilberry fruit contains chemicals known as anthocyanosides, plant pigments that have excellent antioxidant properties. They scavenge damaging particles in the body known as free radicals, helping to prevent or reverse damage to cells. Antioxidants have been shown to help prevent a number of long-term illnesses such as heart disease, cancer, and an eye disorder called macular degeneration. Bilberry also contains vitamin C, another antioxidant."

Anthocyanosides help build strong blood vessels and improve circulation to all areas of the body. They also prevent blood platelets from clumping together, which reduces the risk of blood clots. And they have antioxidant properties (preventing or reducing damage to cells from free radicals). Anthocyanidins boost the production of *rhodopsin*, a pigment that improves night vision and helps the eye adapt to light changes. Bilberry is also rich in tannins, which act as astringents and have anti-inflammatory properties. Bilberries may also help control diarrhea."[36]

Bilberry supports heart and blood vessel conditions, including those associated with atherosclerosis, varicose veins, decreased blood flow in the veins, and chest pain. The fruit has been used in cases of chronic fatigue syndrome (CFS), hemorrhoids, diabetes, osteoarthritis,

---

[34] Milbury, Paul E, Brigitte Graf, Joanne M. Curran-Celentano and Jeffrey B. Blumberg, Bilberry (Vaccinium myrtillus) Anthocyanins Modulate Heme Oxygenase-1 and Glutathione S-Transferase-pi Expression in ARPE-19 Cells, Investigative Ophthalmology and Visual Science. 2007;48:2343-2349, 2007

[35] Duke, PhD, James, *The Green Pharmacy*, p. 45

[36] University of Maryland Medical Center, "Bilberry," Reviewed by Stephen Ehrlich, NMD, 2008

gout, skin infections, gastrointestinal (GI) disorders, kidney disease, and urinary tract infections (UTIs).[37]

---

[37] Bilberry, http://www.webmd.com/vitamins-supplements/ingredientmono-202-BILBERRY.aspx?activeIngredientId=202&activeIngredientName=BILBERRY&source=2, 2009

Brazilian Berry Attacks Cancer Cells

Over the last few years, a Brazilian berry known well to natives has become a worldwide hit. It's called the açaí (pronounced ah-sah-ee) berry and comes from a type of palm tree growing throughout Central and South America.

Açaí contains antioxidants that destroyed cultured human cancer cells in a recent University of Florida study, one of the first studies to investigate the fruit's purported benefits.[38] Published in the *Journal of Agricultural and Food Chemistry,* Stephen Talcott, an assistant professor with University of Florida's Institute of Food and Agricultural Sciences, reported that extracts from açaí berries triggered a self-destruct response in up to 86 percent of leukemia cells tested.

"Açaí berries are already considered one of the richest fruit sources of antioxidants," Talcott said. But he cautioned that the study was not intended to show whether compounds found in açaí berries could prevent leukemia in people. "This was only a cell-culture model and we don't want to give anyone false hope. We are encouraged by the findings, however. Compounds that show good activity against cancer cells in a model system are most likely to have beneficial effects in our bodies."[39]

Other fruits—including grapes, guavas, and mangoes—contain antioxidants shown to kill cancer cells in similar studies, Talcott said. Experts are uncertain as to how much of an effect antioxidants have on cancer cells in the human body because factors such as nutrient absorption, metabolism, and the influence of other biochemical processes may influence antioxidants' chemical activity.

So far, only fundamental research has been done on açaí berries, which contain at least fifty to seventy-five as-yet-unidentified compounds.

"One reason so little is known about açaí berries is that they're perishable and are traditionally used immediately after picking," he

---

[38] Nordlie, Tom, Brazilian berry destroys cancer cells in lab, UF study shows, University of Florida, Gainesville, Jan 06
[39] ibid

said. "Products made with processed açaí berries have only been available for about five years, so researchers in many parts of the world have had little or no opportunity to study them."

Historically, Brazilians have used açaí berries to treat digestive disorders and skin conditions. Current marketing efforts by retail merchants and Internet businesses suggest açaí products can help consumers lose weight, lower cholesterol, and gain energy.

"A lot of claims are being made, but most of them haven't been tested scientifically," Talcott said. "We are just beginning to understand the complexity of the açaí berry and its health-promoting effects."

In the University of Florida study, six different chemical extracts were made from açaí fruit pulp, and each extract was prepared in seven concentrations. Four of the extracts were shown to kill significant numbers of leukemia cells when applied for twenty-four hours. Depending on the extract and concentration, anywhere from about 35 to 86 percent of the cells died.[40]

---

[40] ibid

Pomegranates: Pro-Heart, Anti-Cancer

Pomegranates have been popular since biblical days and were spoken about in Greek mythology. The horticulture department of Perdue University explains the origin of the fruit:

> The pomegranate tree is native from Iran to the Himalayas in northern India and has been cultivated since ancient times throughout the Mediterranean region of Asia, Africa and Europe. The fruit was used in many ways as it is today and was featured in Egyptian mythology and art, praised in the Old Testament of the Bible and in the Babylonian Talmud, and it was carried by desert caravans for the sake of its thirst-quenching juice. It traveled to central and southern India from Iran about the first century A.D. and was reported growing in Indonesia in 1416. It has been widely cultivated throughout India and drier parts of southeast Asia, Malaya, the East Indies and tropical Africa. The most important growing regions are Egypt, China, Afghanistan, Pakistan, Bangladesh, Iran, Iraq, India, Burma and Saudi Arabia. There are some commercial orchards in Israel on the coastal plain and in the Jordan Valley.[41]

Now pomegranates are back in fashion, health-wise. Israeli doctors have discovered that this ancient fruit has antioxidant properties that make it a strong cancer-fighter.

On the heels of this discovery, another Israeli team has found that the fruit could have important implications for breast cancer treatment and estrogen replacement therapy.

The Technion-Israel Institute of Technology research team presented two studies at an international conference in Madrid, Spain, June 2001, indicating that pomegranate seed oil triggers apoptosis—a self-destruct mechanism in breast cancer cells. Furthermore, pomegranate juice can be toxic to most estrogen-dependent breast cancer cells, while leaving normal breast cells largely unaffected.

---

[41] hort.purdue.edu, citing: Morton, J. 1987. Pomegranate. p. 352–355. In: Fruits of warm climates. Julia F. Morton, Miami, FL.

"Pomegranates are unique in that the hormonal combinations inherent in the fruit seem to be helpful both for the prevention and treatment of breast cancer," explains Dr. Ephraim Lansky, who headed the studies. "Pomegranates seem to replace needed estrogen often prescribed to protect postmenopausal women against heart disease and osteoporosis, while selectively destroying estrogen-dependent cancer cells."[42]

Dr. Martin Goldman, a New York-based board certified internist and life medicine specialist, notes, "This is apparently a safe substance that could be helpful to many people, especially women at high-risk for developing breast cancer."[43]

Other research has shown that pomegranate juice is helpful in oxygenating the heart of heart disease patients,[44] combating erectile dysfunction,[45] and fighting prostate cancer.[46] Scientists at Case Western Reserve University have also reported that tissue cultures of human cartilage cells respond to pomegranate extract; inflammation is reduced and the enzymes that break down cartilage become less active.[47]

---

[42] Shayne, PhD, Vic, Nutrition Research Center, Inc., nutritionresearchcenter.org, Pomegranate Seed Oil Causes Cancer Cells To Self-Destruct, *Women's Health Weekly*, Gale Group, Farmington Hills, Michigan September 20, 2001
[43] Novak, Adar, Pomegranate Seed Oil Causes Breast Cancer Cells to Self-Destruct, American Technion Society, August 21, 2001
[44] *American Journal of the College of Cardiology*, Sept. 2005
[45] *Journal of Urology*, July 2005)
[46] *Proceedings of the National Academy of Sciences*, Sept. 26, 2005
[47] *Journal of Nutrition*, Sept. 2005.47

Ginkgo Biloba is a Prized Fighter

Ginkgo biloba is the Rocky Balboa in the world of nutrition, knocking out fatigue, pumping up blood flow, supporting men who have erectile dysfunction,[48] and tackling blood clots in the legs.

The ginkgo tree can be traced back 300 million years and is the oldest surviving species of tree. The Ice Age put an end to the plant in Europe, but it survived in China, Japan, and other parts of East Asia. Ginkgo has been cultivated for ceremonial and medical purposes, and some particularly revered trees have been tended for more than 1,000 years. In traditional Chinese herbology, tea made from ginkgo seeds has been used for an array of health problems, most particularly asthma and other respiratory illnesses. The leaf was not traditionally used, but in the 1950s, German researchers began investigating its medical possibilities in the form of extracts rather than remedies using the seeds.[49]

Doctors at the Mayo Clinic say that in healthy subjects, there's early evidence favoring the use of ginkgo for memory enhancement, altitude (mountain) sickness, symptoms of premenstrual syndrome (PMS), and reduction of chemotherapy-induced end-organ vascular damage.[50]

Dr. Yee Suk Kim and his colleagues at the Catholic University of Seoul in South Korea performed experiments in rats to evaluate the effectiveness of ginkgo against neuropathic pain—a common pain problem associated with herpes zoster, limb injury, or diabetes. The scientists produced the first scientific evidence that ginkgo has a real effect in reducing neuropathic pain, which does not always respond well to available treatments.[51]

---

[48] Becker, MD, Mitchell, Ginkgo Biloba, Part II, Clinical Uses, Brief Clinical Update, UCLA Dept of Medicine, 2009

[49] healthlibrary.epnet.com/GetContent.aspx?token=e0498803-7f62-4563-8d47-5fe33da65dd4&chunkiid=21740

[50] Mayo Clinic, "Ginkgo (Ginkgo biloba L.)," mayoclinic.com/health/ginkgo-biloba/NS_patient-ginkgo, 2009

[51] Ginkgo Reduces Neuropathic Pain In Animal Studies ScienceDaily, (June 12, 2009, citing 2009 June issue of *Anesthesia & Analgesia*, official journal of the International Anesthesia Research Society (IARS)

Working with genetically engineered mice, researchers at Johns Hopkins have shown that daily doses of a standardized extract from ginkgo leaves can prevent or reduce brain damage after an induced stroke. "It's still a large leap from rodent brains to human brains but these results strongly suggest that further research into the protective effects of ginkgo is warranted," said lead researcher Sylvain Doré, PhD, an associate professor in the Department of Anesthesiology and Critical Care Medicine. "If further work confirms what we've seen, we could theoretically recommend a daily regimen of ginkgo to people at high risk of stroke as a preventive measure against brain damage."[52]

In a report on clinical uses of ginkgo, Mitchell Becker, MD, writes, "Many European studies have looked at the effect of Ginkgo biloba extract on peripheral vascular disease. Consistent improvements in patients treated with Ginkgo biloba extract, measured in terms of pain-free walking distance, maximum walking distance, blood flow, transcutaneous (measured across the depth of the skin) oxygen, and decreased blood lactate levels, have all been observed."[53]

While all the mechanisms of ginkgo's healing powers are not known to science, researchers are working to scientifically prove that which traditional uses of the plant have already elucidated—that ginkgo supports mental functions, nerve transmission, and certain types of pain and discomfort relief.

Traditional Chinese physicians use ginkgo leaves to treat asthma and chilblains (inflammation of the small blood vessels in the skin in response to cold—above freezing—temperatures). Ancient Chinese and Japanese people ate roasted ginkgo seeds and considered them a digestive aid and preventive for drunkenness. In the western world, ginkgo grew in popularity since the 1960s when technology made it possible to isolate its essential compounds. Ginkgo's flavonoids act as free-radical scavengers, and its terpenes (ginkgolides) inhibit platelet activating factor. Ginkgo is now one of the most commonly prescribed herbal medications in Europe.[54]

Ginkgo should not be taken while on blood-thinning drugs (including heart medications and aspirin), steroids, or non-steroidal

---

[52] Daily Dose Of Ginkgo May Prevent Brain Cell Damage After Stroke, Mouse Studies Suggest, Science Daily Oct. 10, 2008, citing Johns Hopkins study (2008, October 10). Daily Dose Of Ginkgo May Prevent Brain Cell Damage After Stroke

[53] Becker, MD, Mitchell, Ginkgo Biloba, Part II, Clinical Uses, Brief Clinical Update, UCLA Dept of Medicine, 2009

[54] drugs.com/npc/ginkgo.html

anti-inflammatory medications. This is of special note to the elderly, so don't go out and buy ginkgo for your father or mother without speaking to his or her doctor first.

Ginger's Hope For Ovarian Cancer

Ginger, the age-old root spice, is well-known to midwives and pregnancy experts as the go-to food for nausea. In fact, ginger ale was once sold as a tonic for upset stomach. Chinese medical texts from the 4th century BC suggest that ginger is effective in treating not only nausea, but also diarrhea, stomachaches, cholera, toothaches, bleeding, and rheumatism. Now scientists are finding far more serious problems that ginger can tackle.

If we look inside ginger, scientifically speaking, we find it contains a substance called oleoresin, which drug companies use for digestive, anti-tussive, anti-flatulent, laxative, and antacid compounds. Though called a root, ginger is actually the rhizome of the perennial plant *Zingiber officinale*. Two active constituents of ginger are zingerone and gingerol.

But what can ginger do for the common cold and flu? You may be surprised. In traditional Chinese medicine, hot ginger tea drunk at the first sign of a cold is believed to help avert infection. Now we have some insight as to why. A study led by Dr. Hiroshi Ochiai at the Department of Human Science, Faculty of Medicine, Toyama Medical and Pharmaceutical University, Japan, showed ginger to have an inhibitory effect on growth of the influenza virus. The effect comes about as ginger leads to the production of anti-influenza cytokines. Cytokines are a group of proteins used by the body that allow one cell's communication with another. They're released by many types of cells and are a key part of the immune system, involved in fighting a variety of immunological, inflammatory, and infectious diseases.[55]

Of special note is a report published by researchers at the University of Michigan Comprehensive Cancer Center claiming that ginger causes ovarian cancer cells to die. The way in which the cells died in the study suggests that ginger may not face the problem

---

[55] Ginger does ward off flu: study, Chinese Medicine News, chinesemedicinenews.com/?p=38, citing *The American Journal of Chinese Medicine.* 2006-34(1): 157-69

common to standard cancer treatments, wherein cells become resistant to their medications.[56]

Researchers used ginger powder—similar to the kind sold in grocery stores, only a standardized research grade—to dissolve in solution, and applied it to ovarian cancer cell cultures. The ginger induced cell death in all the ovarian cancer cell lines tested. Moreover, the researchers found that ginger caused two types of cell deaths. One type, known as apoptosis, results from cancer cells dying off in a natural fashion of shortened life cycle. The second type of cell death, called *autophagy*, results from cells digesting (or attacking) themselves.

"Most ovarian cancer patients develop recurrent disease that eventually becomes resistant to standard chemotherapy—which is associated with resistance to apoptosis. If ginger can cause autophagic cell death in addition to apoptosis, it may circumvent resistance to conventional chemotherapy," said study author J. Rebecca Liu, MD, assistant professor of obstetrics and gynecology at the University of Michigan Medical School and a member of the University of Michigan Comprehensive Cancer Center. Study results are preliminary, and researchers plan to test whether they can obtain similar results in animal studies. The appeal of ginger as a potential treatment for ovarian cancer is that it would have virtually no side effects and would be easy to administer as a capsule.

Ginger is effective at controlling inflammation, and inflammation contributes to the development of ovarian cancer cells. By halting the inflammatory reaction, the researchers suspect, ginger should also stop cancer cells from growing.

"In multiple ovarian cancer cell lines, we found that ginger induced cell death at a similar or better rate than the platinum-based chemotherapy drugs typically used to treat ovarian cancer," said Jennifer Rhode, MD, a gynecologic oncology fellow at the University of Michigan Medical School.[57]

Studies on ginger continue to show its potential benefits in fighting heart disease, cancer, diabetes, and inflammation.

---

[56] Liu, MD, Rebecca, Jennifer Rhode, MD, Ginger causes ovarian cancer cells to die, U-M researchers find, Cell studies show promise for ginger as potential ovarian cancer treatment, University of Michigan Health System, Additional study authors were undergraduate student Jennifer Huang, research associates Sarah Fogoros and Lijun Tan, and Suzanna Zick, N.D., M.P.H., research investigator in family medicine. Ap 06
[57] ibid

Biomedical researchers report, "Ginger has been shown to possess anti-diabetic activity in a variety of animal studies. A study found that when rats were given ginger juice for 6 weeks, the risk for developing diabetes was reduced. The researchers found that treatment with *ginger* significantly increased insulin levels and decreased fasting glucose levels. Treatment with *ginger* also produced other favorable effects in diabetic rats, including decreases in serum cholesterol, triglycerides, and blood pressure."[58]

Ginger's active ingredient, gingerol has the potential to stop a cancerous cell from reproducing by blocking a tumor's vessel formation, which cuts off its blood supply.[59] Researchers have shown that ginger-supplemented rats had a significantly smaller number of tumors and cancer incidence.[60]

---

[58] *Pennington Nutrition Series*, Healthier lives through education in nutrition and preventive medicine, Pennington Biomedical Research Center, 2007 No. 6
[59] ibid
[60] ibid

Pau d'Arco: Healing Treasure of the Amazon

It's difficult to find an herb that has so many reported applications as Pau d'arco, from the Amazon rainforest. While natives have used this herb to combat an amazing breadth of health problems, modern science has yet to catch up with them. Still, as you read further, there are several researchers who have worked with Pau d'arco and say that it offers great promise.

Pau d'arco has been used traditionally for colds, flu, boils, chlorosis, colitis, diarrhea, dysentery, enuresis, fever, pharyngitis, snakebites, ringworm, scabies, poor immunity, syphilis, wounds, cancer, ulcers, respiratory problems, arthritis, cystitis, prostatitis, poor circulation, diabetes, rheumatism, constipation, and cancer. [61] [62] This super plant is truly one of the wonders of the herbal arsenal.

To go into all of Pau d'arco's suggested benefits is to reach beyond the scope of this book. Yet, it is of note that beta-lapachone, an active ingredient in Pau d'arco, causes cancer cell death.[63] Lucy Snyder, researcher at the University of Texas, wrote, "Beta-lapachone works by disrupting DNA replication. Topoisomerase I is an enzyme that unwinds the DNA that makes up the chromosomes. The chromosomes must be unwound in order for the cell to use the genetic information to synthesize proteins; beta-lapachone keeps the chromosomes wound tight, and so the cell can't make proteins. As a result, the cell stops growing. Because cancer cells grow and reproduce at a much faster rate than normal cells, they are more vulnerable to topoisomerase inhibition than are normal cells. Beta-lapachone also

---

[61] Taylor, ND, Leslie, Ethnomedical Information on Pau d'Arco (Tabebuia impetiginosa), rain-tree.com

[62] Youzhi Li, Xiangao Sun, J. Thomas LaMont, Arthur B. Pardee, and Chiang J. Li, Selective killing of cancer cells by β-lapachone: Direct checkpoint activation as a strategy against cancer, The National Academy of Sciences, 2003

[63] Lee JI, Choi DY, Chung HS, et al. beta-lapachone induces growth inhibition and apoptosis in bladder cancer cells by modulation of Bcl-2 family and activation of caspases. Exp Oncol. 2006;28(1):30-35.

interferes with the replication of HIV-1, a virus that causes AIDS, thereby slowing the advancement of the disease."[64]

Traditionally, larger doses of this plant have been used to affect major health problems. More study needs to be done on humans subjects. In the meantime, though, if you are thinking about taking Pau d'arco, make sure you have proper health practitioner's supervision.

---

[64] Snyder, Lucy A, "Pharmacology of ß-Lapachone and Lapachol," University of Texas Cyberbotanica, biotech.icmb.utexas.edu/botany/beta.html, May 97

Cilantro's Not Just For Salsa

Cilantro (also called Chinese parsley) is one of the spices that gives Mexican food its great, signature flavor. But did you know it's also used as a potent herb?

Cilantro contains an ingredient called dodecenal, which has been scientifically shown to possess antibacterial qualities. Studies performed by scientists show that cilantro destroys and suppresses the growth and reproduction of bacteria. The fresh leaves of cilantro and its seed, coriander,[65] contain about the same amount of dodecenal.

Researchers believe dodecenal works by destroying the cell membrane surrounding the cytoplasm—a very thin, semi-fluid, sheet-like structure made of four continuous layers of molecules. Dodecenal does not appear to interfere with any of the protein-manufacturing machinery of the cell (as occurs with many commercial antibiotics), so bacteria is less likely to develop resistance to it.[66]

Another recent claim to fame for cilantro is its role in mercury detoxification. Mercury is one of the deadliest metals known to man and exists in cavity fillings (commonly called metal or silver fillings), as well as many fish and pollution. Mercury in the human body leads to mental, neurological, and immunological health problems.

Online health guru Dr. Joseph Mercola writes, "Cilantro mobilizes mercury, aluminum, lead and tin stored in the brain and in the spinal cord and moves it into the connective tissues. The mobilized mercury appears to be either excreted via the stool, the urine, or translocated into more peripheral tissues. The mechanism of action is unknown." Cilantro, by itself, does not necessarily remove mercury from the body; it may just displace the heavy toxic metals intracellularly or from deeper body stores to more superficial structures, where it can be more easily removed by other means.[67]

---

[65] Kubo, Isao, Compound in cilantro may fight bacteria, Department of Environmental Science, Policy and Management, University of California, Berkeley, Food Technology Intelligence, Inc. 05

[66] ibid

[67] Mercola, DO, Joseph, and Dietrich Klinghardt, MD, PhD

Medical Director American Academy of Neural Therapy, mercola.com, citing Ewan KB, Pamphlett R Increased inorganic mercury in spinal motor neurons following chelating agents. Neurotoxicology 1996;17(2):343-349

Astragalus's Potent Immune Benefits

According to researchers at the University of Maryland Medical Center, astragalus (*Astragalus membranaceus*) has been used in Traditional Chinese Medicine for thousands of years, often in combination with other herbs, to strengthen the body against disease. It contains antioxidants, which protect cells against damage caused by free radicals—byproducts of cellular energy. Astragalus is used to protect and support the immune system, for preventing colds and upper respiratory infections, to lower blood pressure, to treat diabetes, and to protect the liver.[68]

Astragalus has antibacterial, anti-inflammatory, and diuretic properties. It's taken internally and is sometimes used topically for wounds. In addition, studies have shown that astragalus has antiviral properties and stimulates the immune system, suggesting that it is indeed effective at preventing colds.

In the United States, researchers have investigated astragalus as a possible treatment for people whose immune systems have been compromised by chemotherapy or radiation. In these studies, astragalus supplements have been shown to speed recovery and extend life expectancy. Research on using astragalus for people with AIDS has produced inconclusive results.

Recent Chinese research indicates that astragalus may offer antioxidant benefits to people with severe forms of heart disease, by relieving symptoms and improving heart function.

---

[68] University of Maryland Medical Center, "Astralagus," Feb 09

Garlic: Spice & Super Food

And then there's garlic—tasty, strong, powerful, and capable of keeping Dracula from your door and out of your basement. This Super Food is so strong that it has been shown to fight cancer and the common cold, as well as to kill bacteria and fungi both topically and in the body!

Garlic belongs to the vegetable family *allium*, which also includes onions, scallions, leeks, and chives. Officially known as *allium sativium*, a member of the lily family that's been a part of the human medicine chest since ancient Egyptian times, Garlic has been traditionally used to treat heart problems, headaches, bites, worms, and tumors. In 1858, French chemist Louis Pasteur reported garlic as having antibiotic properties. In the early twentieth century, Albert Schweitzer used garlic to treat amoebic dysentery. In World War I, garlic was used to prevent gangrene from battle wounds.[69]

Allicin, garlic's main curative component, kills a wide range of bacteria (including drug-resistant strains of E. coli), fungi—particularly *candida albicans* (known better as yeast infection fungi). Garlic is also used against parasites—including some major human intestinal protozoan parasites—and viruses.[70] Garlic's sulfur compounds kill microbes inside your body and on your skin.[71]

Garlic is rich in flavanols, particularly kaempferol, which aid in the detoxification of cancer-causing agents. According to University of Maryland researchers, "A well-designed study of nearly 150 people found that garlic helps prevent and treat the common cold. In this

---

[69] Laboratory: Testing Garlic as an Antimicrobial
Agent, Wilmington College of Ohio,
plato.wilmington.edu/faculty/dburks/BIO231%202009%20%20Garlic%20lab%20for%202009..pdf, 2009
[70] *Microbes Infect.* 1999 Feb;1(2):125-9; Antimicrobial properties of allicin from garlic, Ankri S, Mirelman D, Department of Biological Chemistry, Weizmann Institute of Science, Rehovot, Israel, 1999
[71] Fleishauer, Aaron T and Lenore Arab, Supplement: Recent Advances on the Nutritional Effects Associated with the Use of Garlic as a Supplement, Garlic and Cancer: A Critical Review of the Epidemiologic Literature, Journal of Nutrition. 2001;131:1032S-1040S.) The American Society for Nutritional Sciences, 2001

study, people received either garlic supplements or placebo for 12 weeks during 'cold season' (between the months of November and February). Those who received garlic had significantly fewer colds than those who received placebo. Plus, when faced with a cold, the symptoms dissipated more quickly among those receiving garlic compared to those receiving placebo."[72]

Garlic may be powerful enough to prevent cancer.[73] It's been widely studied for its water- and lipid-soluble allyl sulfur compounds that are effective in blocking myriad chemically-induced tumors. Dr. J.A. Milner, University of Pennsylvania, reports, "The diverse array of compounds and target tissues involved suggests either that garlic or associated constituents have multiple mechanisms of action or, more logically, influence a fundamental step in the overall cancer process."[74]

The American Institute for Cancer Research (AICR) reports, The protective effect of garlic was shown to have a dose response relationship. In other words, highest exposure to the food showed the greatest decrease in risk. For cancer protection, AICR experts suggest including garlic as part of a well-balanced predominantly plant-based diet. These allium vegetables contain many substances now being studied for their anti-cancer effects, such as quercetin, allixin and a large group of organosulfur compounds that includes *allicin, alliin* and *allyl sulfides.* In laboratory studies, components of garlic have shown the ability to slow or stop the growth of tumors in prostate, bladder, colon and stomach tissue. Laboratory research has also shown that one garlic component, called diallyl disulfide, exerts potent preventive effects against cancers of the skin, colon and lung. Recently, this compound proved able to kill leukemia cells in the laboratory."

[72] Ehrlich, NMD, Steven D, University of Maryland Medical Center, 2008

[73] Carlotta Galeone, Claudio Pelucchi, Fabio Levi, Eva Negri, Silvia Franceschi, Renato Talamini, Attilio Giacosa and Carlo La Vecchia, Onion and garlic use and human cancer,[1,2,3] American Journal of Clinical Nutrition, Vol. 84, No. 5, 1027-1032, November 2006, [1] From the Istituto di Ricerche Farmacologiche "Mario Negri," Milan, Italy (CG, CP, EN, and CLV); the Registre vaudois des tumeurs, Institut universitarie de médicine sociale et préventive, CHUV-Falaises 1, Lausanne, Switzerland (FL); the International Agency for Research on Cancer, Lyon, France (SF); the Servizio di Epidemiologia e Biostatistica, Centro di Riferimento Oncologico, Aviano (Pordenone), Italy (RT); the Policlinico di Monza, Monza (Mi), Italy (AG); and the Istituto di Statistica Medica e Biometria, Università degli Studi di Milano, Milan, Italy (CLV)

[74] Milner, JA, Journal of Nutrition. 2001;131:1027S-1031S, Supplement: Recent Advances on the Nutritional Effects Associated with the Use of Garlic as a Supplement, A Historical Perspective on Garlic and Cancer, Nutrition Department, The Pennsylvania State University, University Park, PA, 2001

And in animal studies, components in allium vegetables have slowed the development of cancer in several different stages and body sites: the stomach, breasts, the esophagus, the colon, and lungs.[75]

---

[75] Foods that Fight Cancer, American Institute for Cancer Research, aicr.org/site/PageServer?pagename=foodsthatfightcancer_garlic, Washington, DC, 2009

Quinoa: Aztec Energy Food

If you're looking for more energy, let's take a long trip back in time and journey south of the border. For the last five thousand years, the native peoples of the Andes have eaten quinoa as a staple in their diet. Peoples along the mountain plateaus and in the valleys of Peru, Bolivia, Ecuador, and Chile continue to eat quinoa, which, by the way, means "mother grain" in the Inca language. This crop remains an important food source for the descendants of the Incas, the Quechua, and Aymara peoples (who now live in rural regions).

Quinoa is considered a highly nutritious food by researchers who have discovered that the amount and the quality of protein in its seeds are often superior to those of more common cereal grains.[76] The Food and Agriculture Organization (FAO) of the United Nations has compared the nutritional value of quinoa to that of dried, whole milk.

While quinoa is still used to make flour, soup, breakfast cereal, and alcohol, it's particularly important to note its standing as a Super Food. This is not only because quinoa is rich in vitamins and minerals, but also because it's high in complete protein—"complete" means that it contains all nine essential amino acids needed by the body for a wide variety of functions, from muscle building to new cells growth. Quinoa offers the much-heralded amino acid lysine (needed for tissue growth and repair) and is a good source of manganese, magnesium, iron, copper, and phosphorous.[77]

Ancient South American indigenous warriors referred to quinoa as "the gold of the Incas" because it was so valuable, eaten to

---

[76] E.A. Oelke1, D.H. Putnam1, T.M. Teynor[2], and E.S. Oplinger[3]
1Department of Agronomy and Plant Genetics, University of Minnesota, St. Paul, MN 55108.
[2]Center for Alternative Plant and Animal Products, University of Minnesota, St. Paul, NM 55109.
[3]Department of Agronomy, College of Agricultural and Life Sciences and Cooperative Extension Service, University of Wisconsin-Madison, WI 53706. Feb. 1992; University of Wisconsin-Extension; Alternative Field Crops Manual
[77] Spiridakis, Nicole, Quinoa: A Sacred Super Crop, NPR, National Public Radio, npr.org/templates/story/story.php?storyId=15749697; Oct 31, 07

increase stamina and belonged to a region known for breathtakingly high altitudes and rough terrain. When the Spanish conquered South America, farmers were commanded to stop growing it under penalty of death. Somehow, though, the crop survived and is currently grown in many places, including Colorado.

Quinoa is now prominent in many health-conscious restaurants around the country and sold in health food stores. Quinoa is a natural energy-producer, but unlike other "energy foods," it does not contain caffeine or simple sugars. It does, however, contain some good B vitamins, folate, and whole proteins, which make quinoa reliable as a nutritional means of building energy stores without burdening the body in the way that simple sugars do.

If you suffer from gluten intolerance, you can still eat quinoa; it's considered gluten-free. However, because cross-contamination with non-gluten grains is always possible during processing, it is highly recommended that if you are gluten-free, you buy the products bearing gluten-free designations on their labels. Researchers at Kings College in London suggest,

Quinoa may be a safe alternative for patients with CD [celiac disease]. However, some quinoa products advertised as gluten-free have high levels of gluten [anyway]. Since new legislation to regulate the minimum permitted level of gluten contamination of gluten-free foods is expected to come into place in the near future, further tests will be undertaken to assess the safety of new and existing gluten-free products.[78]

It is noteworthy that "gluten-free" is a relative term, meaning that a product can still contain traces of gluten, yet does not exhibit a gluten-intolerance reaction; and this seems to be where quinoa lies on the scale. Cereal chemists led by researcher C.C. Berti, PhD, state, "The gluten content in quinoa…was less than half that of buckwheat, a pseudo-cereal that already has gained acceptance for use in gluten-free diets." Therefore, "[Q]uinoa could be a safe choice for the production

---

[78] Zevallos, Victor F., L. Irene Herencia, H. Julia Ellis and Paul J. Ciclitira, King's College London, London, UK and 2Universidad Polite´ cnica de Madrid, Madrid, Spain In vitro analysis of gluten-free foods containing quinoa (Chenopodium quinoa Willd.), Summer Meeting 30 June–3 July 2008, Proceedings of the Nutrition Society (2008), 67 (OCE8), E396

of gluten-free products, at least from an immunochemical point of view."[79]

Because it is a good source of magnesium, quinoa may be worth trying if you suffer from migraine headaches. Magnesium relaxes blood vessels, so it also plays a major role in preventing high blood pressure, irregular heartbeats, and cardiovascular disease. Magnesium also acts as a co-factor for more than three hundred enzymes in the body, including those involved in using glucose and in insulin secretion. This is good news in today's high-sugar, highly inflammatory modern diets. Two minerals contained in quinoa serve as co-factors for superoxide dismutase, an antioxidant enzyme that helps protect the mitochondria (energy-producing centers of cells) from oxidative damage that takes place during energy production. Superoxide dismutase also protects other cells, including red blood cells, from injury caused by free radicals.[80]

Quinoa is an ideal energy food to add to your diet, as it helps the cells produce energy. Its vitamin B2 (riboflavin) is a natural energy-producer.

---

[79] Berti, C., C. Ballabio, P. Restani, M. Porrini, F. Bonomi and S. Iametti, Immunochemical and Molecular Properties of Proteins in Chenopodium quinoa, Cereal Chem. 81(2):275–277
[80] http://www.whfoods.com/genpage.php?tname=foodspice&dbid=142

Beets Love Your Liver

It has been proposed that the longevity of rural Russians may be due, to a large part, from eating beets. A mainstay of these centenarians is borscht, a soup made of beets. Whether beets are connected to longevity or not, researchers have found a lot to celebrate in this red root vegetable that benefits the heart, liver, gallbladder, skin, and kidneys. Beets are rich in potassium, iron, magnesium, manganese, phosphorus, and copper, and contain small amounts of calcium, sodium, zinc, and selenium. They also offer vitamin C, folate, and betaine in large quantities. Vitamin A and B complexes are also present in small amounts, as well as traces of beta-carotene.

Because beets are so nutritious, they are a mainstay of detoxification programs, especially when juicing, as part of the regimen. But of the most recent findings for this plant, heart health leads the way with the most benefits. Because they contain nitrates, beets are now reported to help lower blood pressure and benefit athletic performance. By the way, spinach, lettuce, and other green, leafy vegetables also have high levels of nitrate.

In a recent study, volunteers were given either beet juice or water to drink. Their blood pressures were checked by researchers every fifteen minutes for one hour before they drank the juice, and then every fifteen minutes for three hours after drinking it. Researchers also checked every hour for six hours, and then at twenty-four hours after they drank the beet juice. Researchers at Barts and The London School of Medicine reported, "Compared with the water drinkers, blood pressure dropped one hour after the volunteers drank the beet juice. It reached its lowest point two and a half to three hours after ingestion and continued to have an effect for up to twenty-four hours."[81]

It appears that nitrate in the beet juice is converted by bacteria on the tongue into a chemical called nitrite. Once it enters the stomach, nitrite becomes nitric oxide or re-enters the blood stream as nitrite. Apparently, the lowest blood pressure readings occur when nitrite (not nitrate) levels in the blood are at their highest. The nitrites protect

---

[81] Bergman, Elisabeth, Beet Juice Lowers Blood Pressure Nitrates Found in Vegetables May Protect Blood Vessels, WebMD Health News, Feb 08

against endothelial dysfunction, which means that blood vessels have trouble expanding or contracting to handle changes in blood flow. Nitrites also have anti-platelet properties.[82]

If you're a sports enthusiast, or you're getting on in years (who isn't?), you may be pleased to discover that beets are ideal to add to your diet. A new study from the United Kingdom suggests that your stamina can be increased from drinking beetroot juice; you'll be able to exercise for 16 percent longer because the nitrate it contains reduces oxygen uptake, making exercise less tiring. Scientists believe this finding should be of use not only to athletes, but also to elderly people and those with metabolic, respiratory, or cardiovascular diseases.[83]

A constituent of beets is betaine, which carries and donates methyl molecules in the body to help make chemical processes work. Donation of methyl molecules is involved in proper liver function and cellular reproduction. Betaine also helps the body make carnitine, a compound it uses to transport fatty acids to the energy-producing parts of cells. Studies with rats have suggested that betaine may help protect against fatty deposits in the liver, which form with chronic alcohol use, protein malnutrition, obesity, diabetes, and other conditions.[84]

Nutritional pioneers have long lauded the cancer-fighting power of beets, which is why you'll find beets in so many health-promoting juicing recipes. Not long ago, a team of researchers led by University of Wisconsin–Madison food scientist Kirk Parkin showed that beet pigments may boost levels of specific proteins called phase II enzymes that help detoxify potential cancer-causing substances and purge them from the body.[85] In a study published in the *Journal of Agricultural and Food Chemistry*, researchers tested four color varieties of beets: white, orange, red, and dark red. Only extracts from the red beets triggered higher levels of these protective enzymes. The secret is in the pigment.[86]

---

[82] Bergman, Elisabeth, Beet Juice Lowers Blood Pressure Nitrates Found in Vegetables May Protect Blood Vessels, *WebMD Health News*, Feb 08

[83] Paddock, PhD, Catharine, Beetroot Juice Boosts Stamina, UK Study, *Medical News Today,* medicalnewstoday.com/articles/160082.php, Ap 09, citing 6 August issue of the *Journal of Applied Physiology*

[84] University of Maryland Medical Center, "Betaine," umm.edu, 2009

[85] Fischer, Madeline, Beet pigments may help prevent cancer, news.wisc.edu/8108, Dec 2002

[86] ibid

Spirulina, The Super Algae

People living along the shores of Mexican and African lakes have traditionally harvested spirulina plankton for a rich source of food.

Mother Teresa Institute of Health Sciences reports, "Micro-algae are one of the most prolific crops, which represent nearly 90 percent of the photosynthesis on the earth. Spirulina plankton is a blue green vegetable micro-algae found in the highly alkaline lakes of Africa and Mexico. The natives of these places have been using Spirulina as part of their diet for centuries. The only single, natural source providing the highest amount of protein ever known is Spirulina—71 percent. The protein yield per unit area per year is the highest compared to other protein yielding crops. Spirulina provides all essential and non-essential amino acids, all natural vitamins including the "B" complex range and chelated minerals. It contains the highest amount of beta-carotene, a precursor of vitamin-A. It's the only vegetable source of vitamin-B12 and the highest known. The protein content in Spirulina is three times that of soyabean, five times that of meat and vitamin B12, and two and half times that of liver. The amino acid profile of Spirulina protein is similar to that of egg and compared well with food and agricultural organization recommendations."[87]

Strangely enough, the American Society for Microbiology states, "Over the ages, two populations, approximately 10,000 km apart, discovered independently and exploited the nutritional properties of Spirulina. Except perhaps for the Far East, this is the only record of traditional use of a microbial biomass as a food for human consumption."[88]

Spirulina offers a good source of proteins, vitamins, and growth factors, and its linolenic acid (essential fatty acid) content, a

---

[87] Mounissamy, VM, Mother Teressa Institute of Health Sciences, Govt. Pharmacy Building, Gorimedu, Pondicherry; "Wonder gift of nature: spirulina; The Antiseptic, 2002, Jun; 99(6): 193-4

[88] *MICROBIOLOGICAL REVIEWS*, Dec. 1983, p. 551-578 Vol. 47, No. 4; 0146-0749/83/040551-28$02.00/0; Copyright 1983, American Society for Microbiology; Ciferri, Orio, Spirulina, the Edible Microorganism; Department of Genetics and Microbiology, University of Pavia, 27100 Pavia, Italy

candidate growth factor for humans, is also the highest after milk and evening primrose oil. [89]

Modern science has yet to catch up with discovering and documenting all the traditional uses for spirulina. But they do show, thus far, that spirulina is beneficial to animals, as well as to humans.

Spirulina comprises up to 70 percent protein, B-complex vitamins, phycocyanin, chlorophyll, beta-carotene, vitamin E, and numerous other minerals. It contains more beta-carotene than carrots and has been traditionally considered an ideal food for a variety of medical uses, including as an antioxidant, antiviral, antineoplastic, weight loss aid and lipid-lowering agent.[90]

In the fall of 2000, scientists at the University of California discovered that adding spirulina to one's diet boosts the immune system. Immunologists at University of California–Davis School of Medicine and Medical Center cultured immune system cells and found that spirulina increases the production of infection-fighting cytokines (infection-fighting proteins).[91]

They reported, "A number of animal studies have shown Spirulina to be an effective immunomodulator (an agent that can affect the behavior of immune cells.) In rats, spirulina inhibited allergic reactions by suppressing the release of histamine in a dose-dependent fashion, In cats, spirulina enhanced the ability of macrophages [beneficial cells at the site of an infection] to engulf bacteria, and in chickens, spirulina increased antibody responses and the activity of natural killer cells, which destroy infected and cancerous cells in the body."[92]

Eric Gershwin, professor and chief of the Division of Rheumatology, Allergy, and Clinical Immunology at the University of California–Davis said, "Together, increases in these cytokines suggest that Spirulina is a strong proponent for protecting against intracellular pathogens and parasites and can potentially increase the expression of agents that stimulate inflammation, which also helps to protect the body against infectious and potentially harmful micro-organisms. Additional

---

[89] ibid

[90] U.S. National Library of Medicine, Bethesda, MD; National Institutes of Health | Department of Health & Human Services, 2009

[91] UC Davis Study Shows Spirulina Boosts Immune System, University of California, Sacramento, CA, ucdmc.ucdavis.edu/news/spirulina_study.html; Dec 1 00

[92] ibid

studies with individuals consuming Spirulina are needed to determine whether these dramatic effects extend beyond the laboratory."[93]

Spirulina experienced a growth in popularity after it was successfully used by NASA as a dietary supplement for astronauts on space missions.[94] It is currently grown in many countries by synthetic methods. Initially, the interest in spirulina was for its nutritive value: It was found almost equal to other plant proteins. Research suggests it has several therapeutic properties, including cholesterol-lowering properties, immune-supporting properties, anti-viral properties, and a property that reduces the rate of cell mutations.[95]

Spirulina also works as an anti-inflammatory, and multiple studies investigating the effectiveness and the potential of this food in treating several diseases have been performed. A few randomized, controlled trials and reviews suggest that spirulina may improve several symptoms and even have anticancer, antiviral, and anti-allergic effects.[96]

Currently, the consensus is that there needs to be more studies before the benefits of spirulina can be stated without hesitation. In the meantime, the nutrients of this plant food, combined with long-standing traditional use and promising animal studies may be reasons enough to eat spirulina as part of a healthful nutritional program.

---

[93] ibid

[94] Spirulina in Clinical Practice: Evidence-Based Human Applications
P. D. Karkos, S. C. Leong, C. D. Karkos, N. Sivaji and D. A. Assimakopoulos
Department of Otolaryngology, Liverpool University Hospitals, Liverpool, UK, Department of Surgery, Hippocrateio Hospital, Thessaloniki and Department of Otolaryngology, University of Ioannina, Ioannina, Greece

[95] Chamorro G, Salazar M, Favila L, Bourges H., Toxicología, Escuela Nacional de Ciencias Biológicas, Instituto Politécnico Nacional, México, D.F.; Rev Invest Clin. 1996 Sep-Oct;48(5):389-99;

[96] Spirulina in Clinical Practice: Evidence-Based Human Applications P. D. Karkos, S. C. Leong, C. D. Karkos, N. Sivaji and D. A. Assimakopoulos Department of Otolaryngology, Liverpool University Hospitals, Liverpool, UK, Department of Surgery, Hippocrateio Hospital, Thessaloniki and Department of Otolaryngology, University of Ioannina, Ioannina, Greece

Can Kelp Fight Breast Cancer?

Kelp is a form of seaweed rich in iodine and other minerals. In the Far East, especially along the coastal regions, people have been eating kelp for thousands of years, picking it up off the beach and cooking it in their kitchen pots. Now, according to a recent study, there's a question as to whether this seaweed should be added to the arsenal of cancer-fighting foods—especially in treating breast cancer. Some people think that it's the iodine alone within kelp that seems promising. But there's more to think about.

Researchers at the University of California–Berkeley discovered that kelp can reduce the level of hormones related to breast cancer risk. In one study, a diet containing kelp lowered levels of the sex hormone estradiol (the predominant sex hormone present in females) in rats, leading to the hope that it is capable of decreasing the risk of estrogen-dependent diseases in women. The study focused on a type of kelp called bladderwrack, which is closely related to wakame and kombu—the brown seaweeds that are nearly a staple in Japanese cuisine.

Martyn Smith, University of California–Berkeley professor of environmental health sciences and co-author of the study, said, "This study opens up a new avenue for research leading to cancer preventive agents. Kelp is a little-studied nutrient, but there's good reason to look at it more closely."[97]

The study, supported by the National Foundation for Cancer Research and the National Institutes of Health, offers a little more insight into why the Japanese tend to have a relatively low number of cancer cases when compared to the rest of the world.

Prior studies have shown that Japanese women have longer menstrual cycles and lower serum estradiol levels than their Western counterparts, which researchers say may contribute to their lower rates of breast, endometrial, and ovarian cancers. Scientists have been searching Asian diets for clues to the lower rates of cancer, with the

---

[97] Yang, Sarah, New study finds kelp can reduce level of hormone related to breast cancer risk, *UC Berkeley News*, University of California, Berkeley, Feb 05

lion's share of attention being given to soy. But, since soy is not a good addition to the diet (it actually contributes to health problems and hormonal and mineral imbalances), kelp is getting more of the spotlight.

"Brown kelp seaweed makes up more than ten percent of the Japanese diet," said Christine Skibola, assistant research toxicologist at University of California–Berkeley's School of Public Health and lead author of the study.

Skibola said she began the animal study after obtaining encouraging results from earlier case studies of women with highly irregular menstrual cycles.

"The most profound thing I found was that two women with endometriosis and a lot of menstrual irregularities experienced significant improvement in their symptoms after three months of taking 700 milligrams of seaweed capsules per day," said Skibola. "It reduced much of the pain associated with endometriosis and significantly lengthened the total number of days of their menstrual cycles. In one of these women with high estrogen levels, I also saw a drop in blood estradiol levels...after she included kelp in her diet. That led me to believe it was worth doing further controlled studies on kelp."

For the new study, researchers randomly divided twenty-four female rats into three groups. One group was fed a high daily dose of dried, powdered kelp for four weeks, while a second group was fed a low daily dose. Both groups were compared with a third control group of rats that did not receive kelp. To ensure that all the kelp was eaten, Skibola and study co-author John Curry, a University of California–Berkeley post-doctoral fellow in molecular and cell biology, sprinkled the powdered kelp onto apple wedges, one of the rats' favorite foods.

The researchers said the experimental doses of kelp consumed by the rats were roughly equivalent to the amount of brown seaweed eaten by people in Japan. The researchers found that the rats' estrous cycles increased from an average of 4.3 to 5.4 days for the low dose kelp group, and to 5.9 days for the high dose kelp group. Overall, dietary kelp resulted in a 37 percent increase in the length of the rats' estrous cycle.

What does this mean? Studies in humans have linked longer menstrual cycle lengths to lower risk of breast, ovarian, and endometrial cancers. "If you have longer cycles, you actually have fewer periods over a lifetime, which means less time is spent overall in the phases where hormone levels and breast and endometrial cell proliferation are at their highest," explained Skibola.

During the early part of a woman's menstrual cycle, estradiol hormone levels remain relatively constant. Almost halfway through the cycle, estradiol levels surge, peaking just before ovulation. These cyclic periods of high estrogen, which continue over a span of about forty years, from puberty to menopause, stimulate the division of breast cells that already have DNA mutations, as well as increase the chances of developing new mutations—both factors that may increase one's risk of breast cancer.

In a separate test of human ovarian-cell cultures, conducted in collaboration with colleagues at University of California–Davis, dosing with kelp extract led to a 23 to 35 percent decrease in estradiol levels.

"One possibility is that the kelp may be acting as an estrogen antagonist by preventing estradiol from binding with its estrogen receptors," said Skibola. "Our next step is to try to isolate the active compound in kelp that is having this hormone-modulating effect."

Dr. Skibola noted that seaweed contains several complex compounds, including polyphenols, which are considered antioxidants. Kelp supplements are available in health food stores and taken as a source of iodine by people with thyroid conditions.

Aloe and Goodbye to Disease

Aloe vera may very well be the most popular herb/food on the consumer market. You can put it directly on acne to make cysts and pimples disappear, gargle with it for a sore throat, drink some for certain stomach problems, swish it around your mouth for mouth sores and inflamed gums, apply it to sores and wounds, apply it to cracked feet to heal the fissures, and put it on your hair as a healthful gel.

Aloe has been a folk medicine since the days when Cleopatra was trying to coax Anthony into buying her a new necklace.

The University of Iowa's Medical Museum reports,
For over 3,500 years, tales of healing *Aloe vera* plants were passed down by word of mouth. The earliest documented use of *Aloe vera* as a laxative and a treatment for skin problems comes from the ancient Egyptians circa 1500 B.C.E. It was also thought to have been grown and used by King Solomon, who was said to have valued it highly...The Roman naturalist Pliny, writing in the first century C.E., cited many uses for aloe: the fresh juice for external application to heal wounds, bruises, and irritations; and a leaf extract to be taken internally as a tonic, purgative, and jaundice remedy.

When Alexander the Great conquered Egypt, he learned that an island off Somalia teemed with aloes. He immediately seized it to guarantee a supply of the wound treatment for his troops, while keeping the herb from his enemies. Arab traders carried aloe from Spain to Asia around the 6th Century. During his travels in Asia, Marco Polo recorded the various applications of the *Aloe vera* plant. The Spanish Conquistadors noted various herbal medicines in use in Mexico and *Aloe vera* was thought to be the effective agent in many Aztec cures. These medicines were brought back to Europe by the Spanish, during the 16th Century. American pioneers used aloe gel to treat wounds, burns, hemorrhoids and rashes.[98]

The two main components of aloe are its gel (found inside the leaves) and its exudate (found in the juice obtained from the cells

---

[98] University of Iowa Hospitals and Clinics, Nature's Pharmacy: Ancient Knowledge, Modern Medicine,Aloe, Aloe vera, Barbados aloe, Curacao aloe, Iowa City, Iowa, Jun 06

beneath the skin). The gel portion of the plant contains many active constituents, including:

- amino acids
- vitamins
- minerals
- mineral salts
- plant hormones and sterols
- enzymes
- aromatic acids
- polysaccharides

One four-year study of ingested aloe showed prolonged life spans in animal subjects, a decrease in the occurrence and severity of kidney and heart problems, and fewer tumors common to older rats of the breed studied. In a study of aloe on the aging process, performed by Health Science Center faculty at the University of Texas–San Antonio, researchers administered gel from the leaves of the Aloe *Barbadensis* plant to laboratory rats for the duration of their lives.

"There has never been much scientific backup for the ingestion of aloe, although people worldwide use it for medicinal purposes including burns, digestion and as a cathartic (to cause the bowels to move)," said the study's principal investigator, Jeremiah T. Herlihy, PhD, associate professor of physiology. "More people in the world take the gel internally than use it for a skin treatment," he points out, "and we wanted to begin to document what the effects actually are."

According to pathologist Yuji Ikeno, MD, PhD, assistant professor of physiology at the university, who examined the rats after death and found that the pathological profiles of the aloe-fed rats differed significantly from those of the control group in several ways. "The chronic nephropathy (kidney disease) usually found in the Fisher 344 rats at the end of their life span was reduced and so was the cardiomyopathy (disease of the heart muscle)," he reports. He also observed a trend suggesting a slightly lower incidence of neoplastic disease (tumors), as well as a reduced incidence of atrial thrombosis (clot formation in the atrium of the heart), which causes acute heart failure. "Multiple causes of death were reduced, suggesting that the disease burden was lighter in the aloe-fed rats."[99]

---

[99] Lawrence, Mike, Study finds beneficial effects of aloe, UT Health Science Center, University of Texas at San Antonio, Ap 97

While dentists are not particularly known to embrace natural healing substances, some of their researchers recognize that aloe can be used to treat many oral health problems, including canker sores, cold sores, herpes simplex viruses, lichen planus, and gingivitis.[100]

Aloe was studied to help with blood sugar problems. Aloe vera appears "to possess anti-diabetic activity, helping to lower blood sugar and triglyceride levels, which are often high in diabetic patients. Researchers at the Mahidol Medical University, Bangkok, gave subjects one tablespoon of aloe vera juice, twice daily. After only two weeks, blood sugar levels had normalized and triglyceride levels were reduced," according to the trade publication *Natural Products Insider*.[101]

Perhaps one of the most active areas of current scientific investigation is aloe's effect on cancer. According to Gillian McKeith, PhD, author of *Living Food for Health*, "The efficacy of aloe's potent immunostimulant glucomannan has been approved for veterinary use in injectible form for fibrosarcomas and feline leukemia." In one study, forty-four cats, all diagnosed with feline leukemia, were injected with 2 mg of glucomannan weekly for six weeks and reexamined six weeks after termination of the treatment. Three-quarters (77 percent) of the cats were alive at the end of the twelve-week study, which McKeith called significant, as 70 percent of cats will die within eight weeks of diagnosis. The glucomannan from aloe was credited with significant anti-viral, immunostimulant, and bone marrow-stimulating properties by the researchers.[102]

Since early civilizations discovered aloe, the plant has been put to use to help heal wounds and nurture the skin. This is the reason it is in so many skin care products, from lotions to salves. The 1996 *Journal of Alternative and Complementary Medicine* found that aloe vera speeds up wound healing and increases scar strength, perhaps by

---

[100] BioMedicine, Aloe vera: Natural, home remedy treats canker and cold sores citing anuary/February 2005 issue of *General Dentistry*, the Academy of General Dentistry, Richard L. Wynn, PhD

[101] Natural Products Insider, Virgo Publishing, naturalproductsinsider.com/articles/2008/01/the-many-sides-of-aloe.aspx , citing Bunyapraphatsara N. "Antidiabetic activity of aloe vera L juice II. Clinical trial in diabetes mellitus patients in combination with gilbenclamede." Phytomedicine. 1996;3(3):245-8.

[102] Ibid, citing Sheets MA. "Studies of the effect of acemannan (tradename) on retrosirius infections; clinical stabilization of feline leukemia virus-infected cats." Mol Biother. 1991;3(1):41-5

increasing collagen formation. The gel penetrates injured tissues and increases blood flow to the injured areas.[103]

Although aloe has shown significant health benefits, it is not advised to drink it in any great quantity, as it may lead to side effects ranging from mild to serious. It's the opinion of the authors that aloe use should be confined mainly to topical applications on the skin, swished around as a mouthwash, or consumed in very small amounts (no more than an ounce), regardless of what you may read on the Internet. Children and the elderly should avoid drinking aloe unless under the supervision of a doctor.

---

[103] Northwestern Health Sciences University, nwhealth.edu/healthyU/stayHealthy/aloevera.html, 2009

Grape Seeds' Super Secrets

The idea of eating grapes with the seeds intact may not appeal to you, but it is amazing what those seeds can do for your body. Luckily, the seeds can be consumed in supplement form.

The value of grapes has been heralded for thousands of years. The grape (*Vitis vinifera*) has been around for at least a hundred million years (but possibly twice that long) Human beings formed a relationship to the plant in the Neolithic period. Wild grapes were harvested by foragers and early farmers. For thousands of years, the fruit has been harvested for medicinal and nutritional value; its history is intimately entwined with the history of wine.

University of Maryland Medical Center researchers tell us that grapes were an important part of the ancient Egyptians' diet at least six thousand years ago. Several ancient Greek philosophers praised the healing power of grapes—usually in the form of wine. "European folk healers developed an ointment from the sap of grapevines to cure skin and eye diseases. Grape leaves were used to stop bleeding, inflammation, and pain, such as the kind brought on by hemorrhoids. Unripe grapes were used to treat sore throats and dried grapes (raisins) were used to heal consumption, constipation, and thirst. The round, ripe, sweet grapes, were used to treat a range of health problems including cancer, cholera, smallpox, nausea, eye infections, as well as skin, kidney, and liver diseases."[104]

Among other beneficial effects, the active compounds in grape seeds are believed to have antioxidant properties. A recent study of healthy volunteers showed that supplementation with grape seed extract substantially increases levels of antioxidants in the blood. To recap, antioxidants are substances that destroy free radicals—damaging compounds in the body that alter cell membranes, tampering with DNA, and even causing cell death. Free radicals occur naturally in the body, but environmental toxins (including ultraviolet light, radiation, smoke, certain prescription and non-prescription drugs, and air pollution) can increase the amount of them. These damaging particles are believed to contribute to the aging process, as well as to the

---

[104] Grape seed, University of Maryland Medical Center website: umm.edu

development of a number of health problems, including heart disease and cancer. Fortunately, antioxidants found in grape seeds can not only neutralize free radicals, but also reduce (or even help prevent) some of the damage they cause.

Not Bad For a Waste Product

Grape seeds are waste products of the winery and grape juice industry. Depending on the variety of grape, its seeds contain lipids, proteins, carbohydrates, and 5 to 8 percent polyphenols. Polyphenols in grape seeds mainly consist of flavonoids (plant pigments that offer health benefits), including gallic acid; the monomeric flavan-3-ols, catechin, epicatechin, gallocatechin, epigallocatechin, and epicatechin 3-O-gallate; and procyanidin dimers, trimers, and more highly polymerized procyanidins. Too much chemistry to remember? Well, you don't have to. Just remember that grape seed extract is known as a powerful antioxidant that protects your body from premature aging, disease, and decay.

Scientific studies have shown that the antioxidant power of grape seed's proanthocyanidins is twenty times greater than vitamin E's and fifty times greater than vitamin C's. Extensive research suggests that grape seed extract is beneficial in many areas of health because of its antioxidant effect to bond with collagen, promoting youthful skin, cell health, elasticity, and flexibility. Other studies have shown that proanthocyanidins help to protect the body from sun damage; improve vision; improve flexibility in joints, arteries, and body tissues such as the heart; and to improve blood circulation by strengthening capillaries, arteries, and veins.[105]

Colon Cancer Responds To Grape Seed Extract

The journal *Clinical Cancer Research* reported that grape seeds' chemicals significantly inhibit growth of colorectal tumors in both cell cultures and mice. A 44 percent reduction of advanced colorectal tumors in the animals occurred with the administration of grape seed extract. Researchers showed that chemicals within grape seed bind with a cancer cell's proteins that freeze the cell's cycle and force it to self destruct.

---

[105] John Shi, Jianmel Yu, Joseph E. Pohorly, Yukio Kakuda. *Journal of Medicinal Food*. December 1, 2003, 6(4): 291-299. doi:10.1089/109662003772519831.

Professor Rajesh Agarwal, PhD, in the Department of Pharmaceutical Sciences at the University of Colorado–Denver's Health Sciences Center said, "The value of this preclinical study is that it shows grape seed extract can attack cancer, and how it works, but much more investigation will be needed before these chemicals can be tested as a human cancer treatment and preventive."[106]

Agarwal explains that because the skin and seeds of grapes are a rich source of proanthocyanidins—a class of antioxidant flavonoids that remove harmful free oxygen radicals from cells—grape products (juice and red wine) are known for their heart healthy effects, especially for lowering levels of blood cholesterol. And because grape seeds contain higher concentrations of these chemicals, they are widely marketed as a dietary supplement.

In 1999, Agarwal and his team of investigators were first to report that grape seed extract also has chemopreventive activity against skin cancer. Their subsequent preclinical work has shown that the extract also retards growth of prostate cancer cells. In this study, Agarwal tested the extract on colorectal cancer, the second most common malignancy and second leading cause of cancer deaths in America. They exposed two different human colon carcinoma cells to the extract and found a dose- and time-dependent inhibition of cancer cell growth.

"Beneficial effects were correlated with how much extract was used and how long it was used for," Agarwal said.[107]

Eyes, Heart, Bone, and Muscle

Scientists with the *National Institutes of Health* reported that researchers found resveratrol to have a variety of positive effects on age-related problems in mice, in addition to cardiovascular difficulties:

- Resveratrol bolsters bone health as measured by bone thickness, volume, mineral content, density, and bending stiffness.
- Resveratrol reduces cataract formation, a condition found to increase with age.

---

[106] Froelich, Warren, Grape seed extract halts cell cycle, checking growth of colorectal tumors in mice, American Association for Cancer Research, Oct 18, 06

[107] Department of Pharmaceutical Sciences at the University of Colorado Health Sciences Center in Denver

- Resveratrol enhanced balance and motor coordination in aged animals.
- Resveratrol allows humans to live longer lives.[108]

Grape Seeds Kill Leukemia Cells

The American Association for Cancer Research (AACR) reports, "An extract from grape seeds forces laboratory leukemia cells to commit cell suicide, according to researchers from the University of Kentucky. They found that within 24 hours, 76 percent of leukemia cells had died after being exposed to the extract." The investigators discovered the extract activates a protein regulating the means by which cells are supposed to die. (One of the features of cancer cells is that they do not die off, like normal cells do). The study's lead author, Xianglin Shi, PhD, a professor in the Graduate Center for Toxicology at the University of Kentucky, said, "What everyone seeks is an agent that has an effect on cancer cells but leaves normal cells alone, and this shows that grape seed extract fits into this category...."[109] Grape seed extract has shown great promise with other cancers, including breast, colon, and lung cancers, but the University of Kentucky study regards hematological cancers—leukemia, lymphoma, and myeloma—which accounted for an estimated 118,310 new cancer cases and almost 54,000 deaths in America in 2006, ranking these cancers as the fourth leading cause of cancer incidence and death in the U.S.[110]

A University of California–Davis study of the supplement benefits on people with high blood pressure found that grape seed extract lowered blood pressure and cholesterol levels. Conducted by the university's cardiovascular researchers, the study was the first human clinical trial to show the effect of grape seed extract on people with metabolic syndrome,[111] a combination of health problems that increase the risk of heart disease and diabetes.

---

[108] Resveratrol, Found In Red Wine, Wards Off Effects Of Age On Heart, Bones, Eyes And Muscle, ScienceDaily (July 3, 2008)

[109] Grape Seed Extract Kills Laboratory Leukemia Cells, Proving Value of Natural Compounds, American Association for Cancer Research, Philadelphia, PA, aacr.org, December 31, 2008

[110] ibid

[111] Ong, David, UC DAVIS STUDY SHOWS GRAPE SEED EXTRACT MAY BE EFFECTIVE IN REDUCING BLOOD PRESSURE, News from UC Davis Health System, Promising results prompt second human clinical study, University of California, Davis, Sacramento, March 26, 2006

It is estimated that 40 percent of American adults (50 million people) have metabolic syndrome, which is a group of risk factors in one person, including:

- Abdominal obesity (excessive fat tissue in and around the abdomen)
- Atherogenic dyslipidemia (blood fat disorders—high triglycerides, low HDL cholesterol and high LDL cholesterol—that lead to plaque buildups in artery walls)
- Elevated blood pressure
- Insulin resistance or glucose intolerance (where the body can't properly use insulin or blood sugar)
- Prothrombotic state (blood clotting)
- Proinflammatory state (too much inflammation)

The one-month university study involved twenty-four male and female patients diagnosed with metabolic syndrome. Those taking 300 mg of grape seed extract had reduced LDL cholesterol levels.

Three previous studies in animal models by the University of California–Davis research team indicated that grape seed extract may also prevent atherosclerosis.

The Power of Pineapples

The popularity of pineapples is surpassed only by their numerous health benefits. Most people would be surprised to learn that the fruit isn't originally from the South Pacific but is actually native to southern Brazil and Paraguay. The fruit was first domesticated by Native Americans and migrated into South and Central America, to Mexico and the West Indies long before the arrival of Europeans. Food historian Julia Morton writes:

> Christopher Columbus and his shipmates saw the pineapple for the first time on the island of Guadeloupe in 1493 and then again in Panama in 1502. Caribbean Indians placed pineapples or pineapple crowns outside the entrances to their dwellings as symbols of friendship and hospitality. Europeans adopted the motif and the fruit was represented in carvings over doorways in Spain, England, and later in New England for many years. The plant has become naturalized in Costa Rica, Guatemala, Honduras and Trinidad but the fruits of wild plants are hardly edible. Spaniards introduced the pineapple into the Philippines and may have taken it to Hawaii and Guam early in the 16th Century.[112]

The meat of the pineapple is not where all the benefits come from. Scientists recently found that the stems of the fruit contain cancer-fighting molecules. "One molecule called CCS blocks a protein called Ras, which is defective in approximately 30% of all cancers. The other, called CCZ, stimulates the body's own immune system to target and kill cancer cells."[113]

Pineapples are considered healthful for a number of reasons. They are a good source of vitamin C, feature strong enzymes that break down proteins, and aid in digestion. The key ingredient in pineapples, health-wise, is an enzyme called bromelain that offers anti-

---

[112] Morton, J, Pineapple. Fruits of warm climates. p. 18–28, Julia F. Morton, Miami, FL 1987

[113] "Pineapple stem may combat cancer," BBC News, news.bbc.co.uk/2/hi/health/4697739.stm, Jul 05

inflammatory effects known to help with asthma,[114] allergies, skin problems, and immune system disorders.[115] Pineapple's bromelain is useful for injuries (sports and other), arthritis,[116] and other issues involving swelling. It's also helpful for sinusitis, healing after surgery, and digestive problems.

In studying pineapple's bromelain against asthma, one study's researcher, Eric Secor from the National Institutes of Health, Post Doctoral Fellow, found that bromelain significantly reduced the body's total white blood cell count, which typically increases with the onset of asthma. Furthermore, with bromelain treatment, eosinophils (the main inflammatory cells associated with asthma) were reduced by more than 50 percent in the lungs.[117] In layman's terms, this means that bromelain helps with inflammation associated with asthma.

Researchers at Queensland Institute of Medical Research (QIMR) reported the discovery of two proteins in pineapples that are capable of blocking the growth of a broad range of tumor cells, including those in breasts, lungs, the colon, and ovaries.[118]

Pineapple is also an ingredient in many topical skin care formulas. Along with its enzymes, pineapple has other active principles that have a beneficial effect on skin.[119] Among these are sulfur compounds as well as a diverse assortment of esters, hydrocarbons,

---

[114] Pennington, Carolyn, Research on pineapple extract may bear fruit for asthma sufferers, University of Connecticut, Advance Newsletter, Oct 09

[115] Tracey L. Mynott[1,*], Andrew Ladhams[*], Pierre Scarmato[*] and Christian R. Engwerda, [*] Department of Biochemistry, Imperial College of Science, Technology and Medicine, London, United Kingdom, and Cortecs, Clwyd, United Kingdom; and Department of Infectious and Tropical Diseases, London School of Hygiene and Tropical Medicine, London, United Kingdom, Bromelain, from Pineapple Stems, Proteolytically Blocks Activation of Extracellular Regulated Kinase-2 in T Cells, The Journal of Immunology, 1999, 163: 2568-2575

[116] Brien S, Lewith G, Walker A (2004). "Bromelain as a Treatment for Osteoarthritis: a Review of Clinical Studies". Evidence-based complementary and alternative medicine: eCAM. 1 (3): 251–257. doi:10.1093/ecam/neh035. PMID 15841258

[117] ibid

[118] Bitange Nipa Tochi , Zhang Wang, Shi - Ying Xu and Wenbin Zhang, Therapeutic Application of Pineapple Protease (Bromelain): A Review, Department of Food Science and Engineering, School of Food Science and Technology, Pakistan Journal of Nutrition 7 (4): 513-520, 2008

[119] Taussig SJ, Batkin S., Bromelain, the enzyme complex of pineapple (Ananas comosus) and its clinical application. An update. J Ethnopharmacol. 1988 Feb-Mar;22(2):191-203

alcohols and carbonyl compounds. In essence, it's not pineapple's vitamin C and bromelain alone that make the plant so healthful.

On its website, Dole, the company best known for distribution of pineapples in the United States, reports that a study published in Cancer Letters suggests pineapple's bromelain might offer some protection against skin cancer. Indian researchers compared the incidence of tumors in mice predisposed to skin cancer after bathing some of the animals in bromelain. Mice treated with bromelain enjoyed a 66 percent drop in the number of tumors they eventually developed—and even those tumors were 35 percent smaller than they would otherwise have been. Plus, 30 percent of the bromelain group never developed tumors at all (all the mice without bromelain eventually had some skin cancer).[120]

---

[120] dole.com

Healing Potential Hidden In Seeds

The greatest secret a food has is in its seed. Hidden deep inside it is the very essence of life's creation. It's been thousands of years since the beginnings of agriculture and there is still no explanation for that which we call "life force." We do know, however, that seeds contain life-giving nutrients, including vitamins, minerals, important fats, amino acids, etc. Among the many seeds offering wonderful nutrition are those of sunflower, flax, sesame, pumpkin, grape, hemp, and pomegranate. The fats and fat-soluble vitamins in seeds offer nutrition for the brain, nerves, glands, hormonal system, organs, eyes, joints, respiratory system, skin, and lungs.

Sunflower Seeds

Birds started off eating sunflower seeds, and now we see baseball players chewing and spitting out the shells as a replacement for the more repugnant tobacco of olden days. Is it just nervous energy that motivates them, or are athletes feeling the energy contained within those seeds?

Sunflower seeds are rich in nutrients. They contain vitamins A, K, B, and E, as well as choline and the minerals calcium, iron, magnesium, phosphorus, potassium, sodium, zinc, copper, manganese, and selenium. Sunflower seeds are also good sources of omega -3s and -6s. Ninety percent of the fat found in sunflower seeds is unsaturated fat that doctors say help to lower bad cholesterol and maintain good cholesterol in your body. Many nutritionists claim the best whole food source of vitamin E is actually in wheat germ oil. One ounce of sunflower seeds contains 76 percent of the recommended daily allowance. With all this basic nutrition, sunflower seeds are ideal for those suffering with low energy, as well as skin, gland, and organ problems.

Flax Seeds

Decades ago, Dr. Johanna Budwig swore by flax seeds as part of her cancer treatment program. While it is the opinion of this author that there is no guaranteed cure for cancer, there is some valuable nutrition buried within the seed of the flax plant. University of Illinois's

McKinley Health Center reports, "The high lignin content of flaxseed is thought to play a role in fighting a broad range of cancers. The anti-cancer properties of flaxseed may also stem from alpha linolenic acid (an omega-3 fatty acid found in flaxseed), which is potentially capable of slowing tumor growth."[121]

Omega-3 fatty acids are important for maintaining the structure of cell membranes, enabling the transport and use of cholesterol, and regulating the production of genes and enzymes in the body.

University of Wisconsin at Urbana Champaign researchers report:

> Clinical studies have shown that flaxseed may lower triglycerides, total cholesterol, and LDL cholesterol levels and reduce the risk of blood clots when consumed over time. These benefits may result from fiber and/or the alpha linolenic acid found in flaxseed. The anti-inflammatory properties of omega-3 fatty acids have been recognized in both treating and slowing the progression of rheumatoid arthritis and kidney disease. Although most omega-3 research has focused on the omega-3 fatty acids found in fish, more recent studies have shown flaxseeds also may provide this benefit. Lastly, flaxseeds are a rich source of phytoestrogens. Some studies have shown that consuming foods high in phytoestrogens may prevent or mitigate symptoms caused by the declining estrogen levels associated with menopause. Phytoestrogens may also be helpful in fighting osteoporosis related bone loss experienced by some post-menopausal women.[122]

Hemp Seeds

Hemp is one of the most versatile plants known to man. It has nutritional value as well as industrial value. But at some point along the way, due to the power of politics, hemp was banned as a crop and unfairly associated with marijuana. George Washington and Thomas Jefferson grew hemp, and Ben Franklin owned a mill that produced hemp paper. Jefferson drafted the Declaration of Independence on hemp paper, and until the late 19th century, more than seventy-five percent of the world's paper was made with hemp fiber. In 1937

---

[121] University of Wisconsin at Urbana Champaign, McKinley Health Center, "Flax Seeds and Nutritional Needs," 2009
[122] ibid

Popular Science magazine claimed that hemp was 'The New Billion Dollar Crop.' Just as it was on the rise, the use of hemp was criminalized. Newspaper publisher William Randolph Hearst led the crusade to ban the plant and all of its uses in industry and the private sector. As an owner of millions of acres of prime timberland, Hearst saw hemp as a major threat to his empire. A machine that simplified the process of making paper from hemp had been invented, but Hearst used his publishing and political power to create public panic about the evils of the plant and marijuana.[123] He effectively crushed his competition and stunted the use of a plant that would have contributed in myriad ways to a better world.

Here we are, many decades later, and hemp seems to have been set free by a less partial judicial system. Courts have ruled that hemp cannot be considered a drug and therefore cannot be illegal to grow. Thanks to the continuous fight by hemp farmers, what has emerged, among other great products, are foods made from the hemp plant: hemp butter, oil, and protein shakes.

Of particular interest are hemp seeds and oil, which are good sources of omega-3 fatty acids, protein, fiber, and vitamin E.

Hemp seeds contain essential amino acids and essential fatty acids to maintain healthy human life. Although flax and other seeds also contain all essential amino acids, hemp has the highest amount of globulin edistin in the plant kingdom. Globulin is the third most abundant protein in the human body and performs many enzymatic functions. This protein is responsible for natural and acquired immunity against invading organisms. Globulins neutralize alien microorganisms and toxins, which means that eating hemp seeds is a great way to bolster your immune system and stay healthy.[124]

Are We Headed Toward A Seedless World?

On a more human, as well as a more planetary, level, doing away with (and controlling) plant seeds, as is the activity of the Monsanto corporation, will lead to catastrophic consequences, out of the selfish consolidation of agriculture into one hand. *Hemp Line Journal* reports, "Those who control the world's distribution of seeds, control the world's food supply and Monsanto is dominating the global

---

[123] Shirt Magic, Lewiston, CA, altahemp.com/hempinfo.html, 2009
[124] Osburn, Lynn, Hemp Seed: The most nutritionally complete food source in the world, *Hemp Line Journal*, July-August 1992, pp. 14-15, Vol. I No. 1

seed market. It is currently the world's largest seed company, after only a decade of entering the industry."[125]

Joseph Mercola, DO, writes:

There is a reason why I believe Monsanto to be one of the most evil companies on the planet, and this is in large part due to its activities relating to controlling food production through controlling the seeds to produce it. For nearly all of its history the United States Patent and Trademark Office refused to grant patents on seeds, viewing them as life-forms with too many variables to be patented. But in 1980 the U.S. Supreme Court allowed for seed patents in a five-to-four decision, laying the groundwork for a handful of corporations to begin taking control of the world's food supply. Since the 1980s, Monsanto has become the world leader in genetic modification of seeds and has won at least 674 biotechnology patents, more than any other company. Farmers who buy Monsanto's GM seeds are required to sign an agreement promising not to save the seeds or sell them to other farmers. The result? Farmers must buy new seeds every year, and they must buy them from Monsanto. Monsanto is considering using what's known as terminator technology on a wide-scale basis. These are seeds that have been genetically modified to "self-destruct." In other words, the seeds (and the forthcoming crops) are sterile, which means farmers must buy them again each year.[126]

Monsanto was also one of the first companies to start commercially marketing DDT and has also been a major producer of Agent Orange, Roundup, and other toxic chemical herbicides, as well as bovine growth hormone, which forcefully increases milk production in cows.

---

[125] Media Environment, Monsanto: Senseless; The World: Seedless, February 13, 2009,
[126] Mercola, DO, Joseph, Monsanto's Many Attempts to Destroy All Seeds but Their Own, http://articles.mercola.com/sites/articles/archive/2009/03/07/Monsantos-Many-Attempts-to-Destroy-All-Seeds-but-Their-Own.aspx

Don't Mow the Dandelions!

If you have a lawn, you may curse dandelions all your life. But if you could only see the health benefits of this plant! The leaves and roots of the dandelion are used fresh or dried in teas, capsules, or extracts. Dandelion leaves are used in salads or are cooked as side dishes. Their flowers are used to make wine. If you are an ardent juicer, dandelion greens make an excellent addition to your juice, increasing your calcium, potassium, and chlorophyll, among other things.

Herbalists swear by this plant that dots your yard with bright yellow flowers faster than you can mow them down. Dandelions have been traditionally used to improve liver health, treat digestive disturbances, and increase bile flow from the liver and gallbladder to help detoxify the body, stimulate appetite, and relieve skin problems.[127]

James Duke, PhD, writes, "I recommend using both the leaves and the flowers. Dandelion flowers are well-endowed with lecithin, a nutrient that has been proven useful in various liver ailments...Since dandelion is a food plant, I suggest steaming the leaves and flowers like spinach and eating a lot of this delicious vegetable."[128]

Duke also writes, "Dandelion root is a particularly potent diuretic. Diuretics don't cure bladder infections, but they help flush urine out of the bladder, and some bacteria along with it. Long clinical experience suggests that this action is helpful in treating bladder infections....Two groups of chemicals that have been found in the plant, eudesmanolides and germacranolides, appear to play a role. The potassium in dandelion may also contribute to its diuretic effect."[129] Diuretic plants are often used by natural doctors to address inflammation, as well as pneumonia, bronchitis, and other respiratory diseases.

---

[127] Health Canada, Drug & Health Products online, 2009
[128] Duke, PhD, James, *The Green Pharmacy*, p. 310
[129] ibid, p. 83

Olive Leaf's Antibiotic Nature

Modern medicine has gone crazy with its overuse of antibiotics. Antibiotics cause a great number of side effects, including the killing of "good bacteria" in the intestines, yeast overgrowth, yeast infections, and a suppressed immune system. And worse, many forms of bacteria are now resistant to antibiotics.

Fortunately, nature may have the answer: There are many natural substances, foods, and herbs that kill fungus and bacteria. The olive tree is ancient in man's medicinal arsenal. The fruit of the tree—olives—has been eaten for thousands of years, but the leaves are of special interest to anyone looking to kill bacteria and fungi in and on their bodies. Olive leaf extract (OLE) has been shown to be useful with:

- Viruses
- Bacteria
- Fungi
- Colds and flu
- Jock itch
- Vaginal yeast infections
- Nail fungus infections
- High blood sugar
- Heart disease[130] [131]
- HIV[132]
- Cancer[133]

---

[130] Visoli, F, G Bellomo, C Galli, Free radical-scavenging properties of olive oil polyphenols. *Biochem Biophys Res Commun* 1998;247:60-4

[131] Somova LI, Shode FO, Ramnanan P, Nadar A. Antihypertensive, antiatherosclerotic and antioxidant activity of triterpenoids isolated from Olea europaea, subspecies africana leaves. *Journal of Ethnopharmacology*.Vol.84(2-3)()(pp 299-305), 2003. 2003;299-305

[132] Lee-Huang S, Zhang L, Huang PL, Chang YT, Huang PL. Anti-HIV activity of olive leaf extract (OLE) and modulation of host cell gene expression by HIV-1 infection and OLE treatment. Biochem.Biophys.Res Commun. 2003;307:1029-3

[133] Leila ABAZA, Terence P. N. TALORETE, Parida YAMADA, Yui KURITA, Mokhtar ZARROUK and Hiroko ISODA, "Induction of Growth Inhibition and Differentiation of Human Leukemia HL-60 Cells by a Tunisian Gerboui Olive Leaf Extract", Biosci. Biotechnol. Biochem., Vol. 71, 1306-1312 (2007)

Researcher, H.E. Renis, in the journal *Antimicrobial Agents & Chemotherapy*, wrote that olive leaf extract has been shown to be effective against the following microorganisms: *E. coli, Pseudomonas aeruginosa, S. aureus, K. pneumoniae, Trichophyton mentagrophytes, Microsporum canis, T. rubrum* and *Candida albicans.*[134] Researchers have shown that the substances in olive leaf—particularly *elenolic* acid and its salt, calcium elenolate—destroy an array of viruses, including parainfluenza, Herpes simplex, pseudorabies, polio (viruses -1, -2, and -3), rhinoviruses, myxoviruses, coxsackie virus, Varicella zoster, encephalomyocarditis, and two strains of leukemia viruses.[135]

The Die-Off Effect
It's helpful to know that if you're using OLE internally, there's something called a "die-off" effect. This means that when OLE kills off bacteria and fungi, the body will suddenly have to handle the dead substances and their toxic wastes. This may cause temporary effects that can range from headaches to fatigue to rashes to aches. In essence, when the bacteria and fungi die off, you feel worse before you feel better.

There are a few ways to handle the die-off effect: reduce the dosage of the olive leaf supplement, drink a lot of water, or bear it. Many natural health practitioners feel that when the die-off effect takes place and you get the symptoms, then you know you're having success in your treatment.

Side Effects And Interactions
Olive leaf extract expands blood vessels. So if you are on a medication of any kind, discuss your particular needs with your physician. OLE should not be taken along with antibiotics, additional amino acids, or any other mold or fungus derivatives because OLE will see them as foreign invaders and kill them. As with any potent herb, be careful not to take too much or take it too frequently to avoid stress on your liver, as well as other side effects.

---

[134] Memorial Sloan Kettering Cancer Center, mskcc.org/mskcc/html/69315.cfm, citing Markin D, Duek L, Berdicevsky I. In vitro antimicrobial activity of olive leaves. Mycoses 2003;46:132-6
[135] Renis HE. In vitro antiviral activity of calcium elenolate. Antimicrob Agents Chemother (Bethesda) 1969;9;167-172

Olive Oil: When It's Good, It's Good

Before discussing the wonderful benefits of olive oil, here's a statement that may come as a shock to you, though it's true: The olive oil industry is full of fraud—the olive oil you think you're eating may not actually be olive oil, even if the bottle tells you the oil is from Italy, that it's cold pressed, and it's extra virgin.

Fraud Is As Ancient As Olives
In the first century, Roman oil was transported in vessels called amphorae. Each amphora was painted with the weight of its olive oil, the farm where it was grown, the merchant who obtained the oil, and the official who verified the authenticity of the oil. The fear was that unscrupulous merchants might substitute inferior oil en route.[136] Here we are, many centuries later, and the concerns over tampering with good oil have not changed.

In 2010, University of California–Davis conducted a study that analyzed nineteen popular brands of olive oil labeled as "extra virgin." Researchers showed that that nearly 70 percent of imported olive oils—but only 10 percent of Californian oils—failed extra-virgin tests. There were three main reasons the oils failed: they were rancid from age; adulterated with cheaper refined olive oil; or were of poor-quality oils, made from damaged, mishandled, or overripe olives.

Restaurant "Olive Oil" May Not Be Pure Either
Most restaurants use a brand of olive oil that is sometimes referred to by the experts as "supermarket olive oil," which is cheap and adulterated. Worse, restaurants commonly cut their olive oil with canola oil. Many companies infuse cheap oils like cottonseed or soybean oil into their olive oil to cheat consumers.

The sad thing about this is that if you're eating olive oil for your health, what you're being fed instead is tearing down your health.

Health Benefits Of Olive Oil

---

[136] Mueller, Tom, "Letter from Italy: Slippery Business," The New Yorker, Aug 13, 2007

Olive oil in its pure and unadulterated form is a Super Food. It is one of the pillars of the much-heralded Mediterranean Diet that researchers say holds the greatest potential for the lowest disease rates (especially heart disease) and healthiest life.

Pure olive oil is a wonderful source of polyphenols. Research shows that polyphenols lower cholesterol[137] and yield other benefits. Polyphenols are antioxidants that protect the cells from the oxidative damage of oxygen "free radicals" that continually circulate throughout the body.

A Portuguese study of the major antioxidants in olive oil showed that one, DHPEA-EDA, protects red blood cells from damage more than any other part of olive oil. This compound is the major source of the health benefit associated with virgin olive oils, which contain increased levels of DHPEA-EDA, compared to other oils. In virgin olive oils, DHPEA-EDA may make up as much as half the total antioxidant component of the oil.[138]

The Olive Oil Times reports: "The phytonutrient in olive oil, oleocanthal, mimics the effect of ibuprofen in reducing inflammation, which can decrease the risk of breast cancer and its recurrence. Squalene and lignans are among the other olive oil components being studied for their possible effects on cancer....It has been demonstrated that a diet that is rich in olive oil, low in saturated fats, moderately rich in carbohydrates and soluble fiber from fruit, vegetables, pulses and grains is the most effective approach for diabetics. It helps lower 'bad' low-density lipoproteins while improving blood sugar control and enhances insulin sensitivity."[139]

Olive oil is a great source of good fats and vitamin E and is rich vitamins A, B-1, B-2, C, D, E, and K , as well as in iron. For thousands of years, olive oil has been used by native Mediterranean cultures as a curative food. Now it is recognized in fighting and/or preventing depression, cancer, osteoporosis, heart disease, strokes, arthritis, high blood pressure, and obesity.

---

[137] Ann Intern Med. 2006 Sep 5;145(5):333-41, *The effect of polyphenols in olive oil on heart disease risk factors: a randomized trial.* Covas MI, Nyyssönen K, Poulsen HE, Kaikkonen J, Zunft HJ, Kiesewetter H, Gaddi A, de la Torre R, Mursu J, Bäumler H,Nascetti S, Salonen JT, Fitó M, Virtanen J, Marrugat J; EUROLIVE Study Group.
[138] Wiley-Blackwell (2009, April 1). Source Of Major Health Benefits In Olive Oil Revealed.
[139] *The Olive Oil Times,* Olive Oil Health Beneftis, Feb 3, 2012

An Uninformed Buyer May Not Recognize Good Oil

Good olive oil gives off a slight burning sensation in the back of the throat. The burning is a sign of the oil's high polyphenol count. Unfortunately, because we are so out of touch with the growing, harvesting, and creation of food these days, few people understand how good oil is supposed to taste.

How Do You Know Which Olive Oil To Buy?

Read the book *Extra Virginity* by Tom Mueller to understand the length and breadth of the olive oil fraud problem. Then you can go online and read up. The more educated you are, the better chances you'll find the real thing and be eating for health.

Olive Growers Who Do Things Right

The website of the California Olive Oil Counsel provides some reliable olive oil sources. One such source is olive grower and producer Albert Katz of KATZ (katzfarm.katzandco.com).

Albert Katz, whose family produces olive oil near Napa Valley, California, and has won twenty-four gold medals over the last ten years for their oil, said, "I was a chef for the first half of my working life and I fell in love with olive oil in the 80's. After a trip to Italy in 1990, I became addicted to the green elixir and vowed that I would come back to California and figure out how to produce it. It has been over 20 years since that trip, but I think I finally have attained that dream."

Regarding the integrity of olive oil on the market today, Katz explained,

> The fact is that Americans in general do not really understand that 'extra virgin' as used by most of the industrial brands found in supermarkets throughout the US means absolutely nothing and is not policed by any federal agency. As you might know, most oils labeled with this designation are not actually EVO (extra virgin oil) even measured against commonly accepted world standards. In fact, studies have shown that close to 80% of those industrial brands are not even made with olives! We have seen a dramatic increase in consumer awareness and education over the last 5-10 years and the proof is in the pudding...so to speak...as we sell out every drop of oil we can produce from our trees every year. So we know many 'enlightened' consumers actually get it!

Apples Take a Bite Out of Cancer

Apples are widely known as a great source of soluble and insoluble fiber. The apple is the ultimate, time-tested Super Food that promises to keep the doctor away. The fruit's soluble fiber helps prevent cholesterol buildup in the lining of blood vessel walls, as in cases of atherosclerosis and heart disease. Insoluble fiber also provides bulk in your intestinal tract, holding water to cleanse and move food quickly through your digestive system.

It is a good idea to eat apples unpeeled because almost half of the vitamin C content is on the underside of its skin. Plus, this is where you get most of the fruit's insoluble fiber. Most of an apple's fragrance cells are also concentrated in the skin, and as it ripens, its skin cells develop more aroma and flavor, a sign that the fruit is at the peak of its nutritional value.

And remember that apples are most healthful when they're organic or biodynamic. As reported by the BBC-reported research conducted by Washington State University–Pullman: "Growing apples organically is not only better for the environment than other methods but makes them taste better than normal apples. Ratios of soluble solids (sugar) content to acidity (tartness), an indication of sweetness, were most often highest in organic fruit. 'These data were confirmed in taste tests by untrained sensory panels that found the organic apples to be sweeter after six months of storage than conventional apples, and less tart at harvest and after six months' storage than conventional and integrated apples.'"[140]

Cancer-Fighting Properties

Phytochemicals in apples help protect against cancer.[141] According to an article published in the scientific journal *Nature*, Cornell associate professor of food science Rui Hai Liu and his colleagues credited phytochemicals—with their antioxidants—in natural apples with inhibiting human liver and colon cancer cell growth. They explain that

---

[140] Kirby, Alex, "Organic apples tickle tastebuds," BBC News, Apr 01
[141] "Disease-fighting chemicals in apples could reduce the risk of breast cancer, Cornell University, Mar 05

antioxidants help prevent cancer by mopping up cell-damaging free radicals and inhibiting the production of reactive substances that could damage normal cells.

"Studies increasingly provide evidence that it is the additive and synergistic effects of the phytochemicals present in fruits and vegetables that are responsible for their potent antioxidant and anticancer activities," Liu said.

"Our findings suggest that consumers may gain more significant health benefits by eating more fruits and vegetables and whole grain foods than in consuming expensive dietary supplements, which do not contain the same array of balanced, complex components," Liu said.

Liu notes that the thousands of phytochemicals in foods vary in molecular size, polarity, and solubility, which could affect how they are absorbed and distributed in different cells, tissues, and organs. "This balanced natural combination of phytochemicals present in fruits and vegetables cannot simply be mimicked by dietary supplements," he explains. "We found that tumor incidence was reduced by 17, 39 and 44 percent in rats fed the human equivalent of one, three or six apples a day, respectively, over 24 weeks."[142]

---

[142] Antioxidant activity of fresh apples. Eberhardt MV, Lee CY, Liu RH Department of Food Science, Cornell University, Ithaca, New York 14853-7201, USA. PMID: 10879522 *Nature* 2000 Jun 22;405(6789):903-4

The Versatility of Calcium Foods

Calcium is the most abundant mineral in the body and is involved in millions of biochemical functions. Because it is a positively charged mineral, it's essential for muscle function, heart health, and fighting fever. The average body contains two to three pounds of calcium, with most of it found in the bones and teeth. While calcium is needed to form bones and teeth, it is also required for blood clotting, transmission of signals in nerve cells, and muscle contraction.[143]

Calcium Plays An Important Role In:
- Cementing skin cells together in cases of cold sores, lip sores, mouth ulcers, and the so-called Herpes virus[144]
- Healing torn tissue from accidents, surgery, nutritional deficiencies, and trauma to the body
- Conducting nerve transmission throughout the entire body, including the heart and other vital organs
- Musculoskeletal function (including muscle response, flexing, and relaxation)
- Bone health and density, preventing osteoporosis
- Fighting infection, by stimulating white blood cell response
- Fighting fever
- Maintaining tooth and gum health
- Supporting hormonal function
- Combatting most types of illnesses
- Preventing hypoparathyroidism, osteomalacia, and rickets
- Treating tetany (muscle spasms) caused by insect bites, sensitivity reactions, cardiac arrest, lead poisoning, and impaired nerve transmission to muscle
- Providing an antidote to magnesium poisoning

---

[143] "Calcium," The Natural Pharmacy: Complete Home Reference to Natural Medicine, 2003
[144] Human Physiology, Wikibooks, can.baidu.com/gangstaliu/snap/14d60942ec38f7c2ae23938d.html; Oct 07

- Preventing muscle cramps in some people
- Acting as an antacid
- Helping to regulate heartbeat
- Treating neonatal hypocalcemia
- Promoting storage and release of some body hormones
- Lowering phosphate concentrations in people with chronic kidney disease
- Preventing high blood pressure

Do You Need Extra Calcium?

Most of us need more calcium if we're not eating a pure diet with a lot of green, leafy vegetables. People who are allergic or who find it difficult to tolerate milk and milk products are said to be missing out on a potential source of calcium, though dairy is not a requirement of good nutrition. People—women especially—who are fifty five years old or older generally need more calcium. Throughout adult life, and especially in periods of pregnancy and lactation, women (as well as drug or alcohol abusers) require additional calcium.

Since calcium is used up during the healing process of tissues, people with chronic wasting illness, excess stress for long periods of time, who undergo surgery, or who have had portions of their gastrointestinal tracts surgically removed need more calcium. People with severe burns or injuries need more calcium, too. Calcium is required by the body in all instances of damages to tissue, from herpes sores to broken bones.

Researchers at the University of Pittsburgh Medical Center report, "According to a large and well-designed study published in a 1998 issue of *American Journal of Obstetrics and Gynecology,* calcium supplements are a simple and effective treatment for a wide variety of PMS symptoms."[145] Symptoms in this study included mood swings, headaches, food cravings, and bloating.

---

[145] "Calcium," University of Pittsburgh Medical Center, upmc.com, 2009

Food Minerals Balance Blood Pressure

High blood pressure rarely has only one cause. Plus, from person to person, the cause may be different. Certainly, there are markers such as overweight conditions, smoking, and arterial disease. Some researchers have pointed to nutritional deficiencies as likely culprits and have looked into calcium's role in combatting hypertension (high blood pressure).

One report from Colorado State University shows that "People with a low calcium intake seem to be at increased risk for hypertension."[146]

"Manipulations of dietary calcium have been repeatedly shown to alter blood pressure in animal models of human essential hypertension. Supplemental dietary calcium lowers blood pressure, whereas restricted calcium diets tend to elevate blood pressure. The mechanisms responsible have not been identified, but numerous possibilities have been proposed. Many of the proposals have attempted to relate dietary calcium to calcium metabolism in vascular smooth muscle and altered vascular tone. Other proposals have focused on neural, hormonal, and renal effects of dietary calcium."[147]

More than eighty studies have reported lowered blood pressure after increasing dietary calcium. Also, calcium-regulating hormones have been found to have an affect on the cardiovascular system and therefore may influence blood pressure.[148]

Some Facts About Minerals And How They Interact To Affect Blood Pressure:

---

[146] Anderson, J., L. Young and E. Long, Colorado State University, "Diet and Hypertension," Nutrition Resources, 2007, no. 9.318

[147] Hatton DC, Yue Q, , McCarron DA., Division of Nephrology, Hypertension, and Clinical Pharmacology, Oregon Health Sciences University, Portland; Mechanisms of calcium's effects on blood pressure; National Library of Medicine; National Institutes of Health

[148] Dietary calcium and blood pressure in experimental models of hypertension. A review; Hatton DC, , McCarron DA.; Division of Nephrology and Hypertension, Oregon Health Sciences University, Portland

- Potassium has an important role in blood pressure treatment because it helps balance sodium in the kidneys.
- Low calcium intake may increase risk of hypertension.
- Excessive sodium intake is linked with high blood pressure in some people.

Dietary recommendations suggest avoidance of too much sodium. The suggested range is 1,100 to 3,300 mg per day. (Table salt is 40 percent sodium. One teaspoon has about 2,000 mg sodium.)

In the United States, hypertension affects one in four adults. Another 25 percent of adults has blood pressure readings considered to be higher than normal. Vegetables, fruits, and dairy products help normalize blood pressure because they're high in electrolytes (naturally-occurring minerals such as potassium, magnesium and calcium).

Theodore A. Kotchen, MD, Professor of Medicine (Endocrinology) at the Medical College of Wisconsin, said studies have shown that individuals eating diets high in potassium—which includes foods such as bananas, dates, potatoes, and raisins—tend to have lower blood pressure.[149]

Paul Rosch, MD, American Institute of Stress, reports, "The first advice generally given to all patients with high blood pressure is to significantly restrict sodium [salt] intake. However, the vast majority fails to respond to this unless they have certain genetic traits. In some, calcium deficiency can be the culprit and they improve with calcium supplementation. These individuals may actually worsen on a low sodium regimen since this would sharply reduce the intake of dairy products that are the major source of dietary calcium. Others benefit from potassium and/or magnesium supplements."[150]

---

[149] Healthlink; Medical College of Wisconsin, "Using Diet to Lower Your Blood Pressure," 2006

[150] Rosch, M.D., Paul J., "Do You Have a Good Blood Pressure?," Health and Stress newsletter (July) of The American Institute of Stress, 2003

Iron-Clad Foods Build Blood

There are two main problems related to iron deficiency: The first is not getting enough iron in the diet. The second is not absorbing the iron that is already present. If you're not absorbing what you have, the solution isn't that you should just ingest more.

Iron is a mineral found in every cell of the body and is considered essential because it's needed to make blood cells. Iron is also a key ingredient in many of the body's proteins, such as the oxygen-carrying proteins called hemoglobin (in red blood cells) and myoglobin (in muscles).

The best food sources of iron include dried beans, dried fruits, whole grains, eggs, liver, red meat, oysters, poultry, salmon, and tuna. Reasonable amounts of iron are also found in lamb, pork, and shellfish.

You can see how, judging by the amount of animal products in list above, vegetarians and vegans may become iron deficient, especially since the iron from vegetables, fruits, grains, and supplements is harder for your body to absorb. Non-animal sources of iron include dried fruits, such as prunes, raisins, and apricots; legumes, including lima beans, soy beans, peas, and kidney beans; almonds and Brazil nuts; vegetables, such as broccoli, spinach, kale, collards, asparagus, and dandelion greens; and whole grains, including wheat, millet, oats, and brown rice.

By adding lean meat, fish, or poultry to beans or dark, leafy greens at a meal, you can improve the absorption of iron from vegetable sources up to three times. Foods rich in vitamin C also increase iron absorption. Some foods, like tea, reduce iron absorption. Black and pekoe teas contain substances that bind to iron, thus rendering it unavailable to your cells.

Your body retains a certain amount of iron in storage to replace any that is lost. But, low iron levels over a long period of time can lead to iron deficiency anemia and worse. Symptoms include lack of energy, shortness of breath, headache, irritability, dizziness, or weight loss. A standard blood test can be used to determine the presence of an iron deficiency.

More than two billion people worldwide are severely affected by iron deficiency, making it one of the leading risk factors for disability and death.[151]

---

[151] Zimmermann, M, R. Hurrell"Nutritional iron deficiency," The Lancet , Volume 370, Issue 9586 , Pages 511 - 520

Nutritional iron deficiency may exist when you can't absorb enough iron from your diet. Researchers have especially noted this by studying populations that eat monotonous plant-based diets. The high rate of iron deficiency in the developing world affects more than just the functioning of individuals' cells; it has greater implications such as substantial health and economic costs, unfavorable pregnancy outcome, impaired school performance, and decreased productivity.

Note: Keep iron supplements away from children—even a little excess iron can be fatal.

K Stands For Bones?

Vitamin K isn't high on the list of "popular" vitamins, but it is crucial to the health of bones and blood. The "K" actually stands for *koagulation*, meaning "coagulation" in Dutch, its discoverer's native language. Henrik Dam was studying the cholesterol metabolism in chicks when he realized that a food factor was influencing blood clotting (coagulation), anemia, and hemorrhaging.

While most doctors tend to look mainly to calcium for building and repairing bones, vitamin K also plays an essential role in bone formation. This is a key factor in osteoporosis as well, where vitamin K is often overlooked as an important nutrient in the daily diet, particularly of older women.

"Making sure a woman's diet contains adequate amounts of vitamin K may help prevent bone loss," reads a study in the *American Journal of Clinical Nutrition*.[152] This study supports previous research indicating that low dietary vitamin K intake is associated with an increased risk of hip fracture. The *Journal* reported in 2003:

In the new study, vitamin K intake was assessed, using a food-frequency questionnaire, in 1,112 men and 1,479 women (average age, 59 years). Women in the study consuming the least amount of vitamin K (25th percentile or lower) had significantly lower bone mineral density of the hip and spine, compared with women eating the most vitamin K (75th percentile or higher). Among the men, there was no association between vitamin K intake and bone density.[153]

Vitamin K is required for the production of a structural protein in bone called *osteocalcin*, which serves as the matrix upon which mineral crystals form in the process of laying down new bone. Without adequate vitamin K, osteocalcin cannot be produced, and bone formation becomes impaired....Studies have shown that women with osteoporosis have significantly lower blood levels of vitamin K, compared with women of the same age who have normal bones. In addition, when women with osteoporosis take supplemental vitamin K,

---

[152] American Journal of Clinical Nutrition. (2003; 77: 512-6).
[153] ibid

the urinary excretion of calcium falls by about 50 percent, suggesting that less calcium is being leached from the bones.[154]

Osteoporosis is a disease in which bones slowly deteriorate until they're thin, porous, and much more likely to break. This increased risk of breaking bones is especially evident in the elderly, which explains the propensity for hip fractures. Some statistics show that a third of all post-menopausal women in the United States develop osteoporosis, resulting in more than a million bone fractures every year.155 Osteoporosis is viewed as mainly a female condition, though men aged eighty or older are greatly affected as well.

Vitamin K is abundant in green vegetables such as peas, lettuce, asparagus, Brussels sprouts, broccoli, spinach, and kale. It is also present in some oils such as sunflower oil, olive oil, and soybean oil. Grain and animal products have very low levels of vitamin K, though higher amounts can be found in organic butter.

---

[154] Gaby, MD, Alan, HealthNotes Newswire (3/27/03)
[155] ibid

Eliminating High-Allergy Foods

Ninety percent of all food allergies are caused by about ten foods. That's the word from the Institute of Food Research in Great Britain.[156] Among the most common allergy-causing foods are fish and fruit. And the culprits within these foods, the substances that cause allergic reactions, are certain types of proteins. In fish allergies, the protein responsible for the reaction is *parvalbumin*; in fruit allergies, it is the *lipid transfer protein* (LTP).

The Top 10 Allergy-Causing Foods Are:
1. Milk
2. Eggs
3. Peanuts
4. Tree nuts (walnuts, cashews, etc.)
5. Fish
6. Shellfish
7. Soy
8. Wheat
9. Tomatoes
10. Corn

In highly allergic people, even minuscule amounts of a food allergen (for example, 1/44,000 of a peanut kernel) can evoke an allergic reaction. Less sensitive people, however, may be able to tolerate relatively larger amounts of a food to which they are allergic.[157]

Melissa Stöppler, MD, in the medical journal *Food Allergy,* wrote, "The allergens in food are those components that are responsible for inciting an allergic reaction. They are proteins that usually resist the heat of cooking, the acid in the stomach, and the intestinal digestive enzymes. As a result, the allergens survive to cross the gastrointestinal lining, enter the bloodstream, and go to target organs, causing allergic

---

[156] Institute of Food Research, Scientists developing food allergy treatment, Feb 09
[157] Stöppler, Melissa Conrad, MD, Food Allergy, medicinenet.com, Feb 09

reactions throughout the body. The mechanism of food allergy involves the immune system and heredity."[158]

---

[158] ibid

Toxins May Cause Weight Problems

A number of doctors have proposed that toxins in our bodies can contribute to overweight conditions. It's good to know that there are many Super Foods that get rid of toxins; help speed up your metabolism; and kill bacteria, yeast, fungi, and viruses.

What are toxins? Toxins are poisons acquired or created from either endogenous (inside your body) or exogenous (outside your body) sources. Endogenous toxins are created by the natural processes of digestion and the cellular metabolic processes that produce body waste. If we do not get these out of our bodies through natural means of elimination, then we'll likely become overwhelmed and sick. Exogenous toxins come in the forms of environmental pollution, artificial ingredients, refined sugar, hair spray chemicals, cosmetic chemicals, pesticides, and artificial fertilizers on foods, prescription drugs, fumes, and so forth. All of these cause more health problems than you may realize.

"[T]he levels of certain substances—synthetic organic/inorganic chemicals—in the environment have coincided with the increasing incidence of obesity that has been documented. These substances are known to damage many of the mechanisms involved in weight control," wrote Dr. Paula Baillie-Hamilton in her study on chemical toxins and obesity.[159] Among these toxins are heavy metals, plastics, medicines, organophosphates, pesticides, and more.

Is It Fat Or VAT?
Eating too much can lead to high insulin levels—the pancreas is made to work harder than normal to remove sugars from your bloodstream and maintain proper balance. If there are too many carbohydrates, or sugars, insulin moves them into your cells where they are stored as fat.

---

[159] Baillie-Hamilton, MB, BS, DPhil, Paula F, Chemical Toxins: A Hypothesis to Explain the Global Obesity Epidemic, The Journal of Alternative and Complementary Medicine, Volume 8, Number 2, 2002, pp. 185–192, Mary Ann Liebert, Inc.

And a major complication that can occur is that your cells can become resistant to the efforts of insulin that's trying to do its job. This is how diabetes develops. Trying to deal with sugar creates a lot of stress on your body, which raises certain hormone levels. And this leads to the accumulation of something called VAT, the fat inside your body, surrounding all your organs: your kidneys, liver, spleen, pancreas, and intestines.

The problem with stress is that it's a push-pull phenomenon. You get stressed, then you become stressed over the fact that you are stressed. This can lead to anxiety, low self-esteem, mental exhaustion, sleepless nights, headaches, ulcers and/or depression. And it certainly leads to eating more comfort foods and sweets in an effort to feel better. This causes even *more* damage to your body and mind. Depression is often influenced by poor or inadequate dietary choices, despite what any psychiatrist may say. While comfort foods may calm people down short-term, they may lead to abdominal obesity if this becomes a long-term dietary pattern. Chronic stress affects important hormones that contribute to VAT deposition.[160]

Toxins Get In The Way
Toxins interfere with your body's natural way of burning fat, creating energy, producing hormones, pumping blood, breathing, and eliminating wastes.

The good news is that you can choose not to eat foods with artificial ingredients. Just read the labels on food packages, and don't eat anything that has chemical names you don't understand. It's that simple: Chemicals are not foods, so don't eat them. It also helps enormously if you avoid eating any foods that aren't organically or biodynamically grown. If your food store doesn't sell organic foods, then pressure the manager to start selling them, or else find a more healthful place to shop. If this fails, go online or find an organic co-op in your area. At home, read the labels of your personal care products—from makeup to deodorant—and get rid of all the ones that list chemicals as ingredients. Artificial chemicals build up in your body and, in addition to making it impossible for you to lose weight, frequently lead to cancer and other diseases.

---

[160] Freedland, Eric S, Role of a critical visceral adipose tissue threshold (CVATT) in metabolic syndrome: implications for controlling dietary carbohydrates: a review, BioMed Central, Nutrition & Metabolism 2004, 1:12 doi:10.1186/1743-7075-1-12, Boston University School of Medicine, Marblehead, MA, Nov 5 2004,

Regarding endogenous toxins, the key is to eat the kinds of foods that help your body process wastes faster and more efficiently, as well as to give your body the energy it needs to do its work. If your body is continually struggling to push out toxic wastes, its energy resources are being drained and there's less of an effort to be made in keeping your cells healthy. Fortunately, there are many Super Foods that help you achieve these goals of losing weight, processing toxins, removing poisons, and creating internal energy within your cells. As you continue to read, you'll discover a number of foods you can easily add to your diet.

Pain Relief with Foods

Pain is a sign from your body telling you there is a problem. While this may sound obvious, consider that if you just get rid of the sign, you may not discover what the problem is until it's too late. Or you may ignore the pain and further injure the affected tissues. This is why so many natural healthcare practitioners recommend quieting the pain at the same time as they treat the underlying problem causing your headache, arthritis, tendonitis, toothache, or sinus pressure, for example.

Of course, there are many degrees of pain. But, generally speaking, pain is most commonly treated by medical doctors with drugs like aspirin, acetaminophin, and even morphine. There are a number of natural approaches to pain that are worth considering for acute and chronic conditions, whether following an accident, surgery, strains, sprains, or an onset of disease. And because most pain is associated with inflammation, it's helpful to allow the body to move through inflammation and repair stages by giving it the nutrients it needs for these biochemical processes. This may be accomplished whether you are taking drugs for pain relief or not. However, it is always wise to coordinate any supplementation with your doctor so that you avoid contraindications (conflicts with prescription medications).

While some foods may help with pain directly (cherries, for example), others help by increasing blood flow to the affected area, such as foods and herbs that dilate blood vessels and support circulation. Hawthorne berries and kudzu are two examples.

Some types of pain—headaches, joint stiffness, neck problems, indigestion, sinus congestion, earaches, stomachaches, etc.—may be caused by eating certain foods (as well as non-foods). Many inflammatory problems are created by arachidonic acid, a type of fatty acid that's natural but causes adverse reactions in some people. This particular pain can be reduced or eradicated by eliminating dietary fats in meat, fish, dairy products, and eggs.[161]

Other sources of pain result from ingesting environmental toxins, drugs (prescription and "recreational"), tobacco smoke,

---

[161] Barnard, MD, Neal; Foods That Fight Pain

pollution, gases, artificial ingredients that constrict blood vessels (MSG, etc.), allergic reactions, food intolerance, obstructions (blockages in blood vessels, the colon, etc.), and a host of irritants, as well as psychological factors. Plus, pain could also be triggered by hormonal imbalances, nerve damage, tooth decay, stress, eyestrain, or physical over-exertion.

Natural Modalities For Pain:
- Acupuncture and acupressure
- Massage
- Chiropractic
- Traditional Chinese medicine
- Yoga
- Tai Chi
- Water therapy
- Exercise
- Coffee (three cups of organic caffeinated will take away many headaches, but beware of the side effects)
- Ice/cold compresses[162]
- Psychotherapy (many instances of pain have a psychological basis)

Some Foods That Help with Pain:
1. Tart cherries
2. Omega-3 fatty acid foods (salmon, mackerel, halibut, and tuna)
3. Ground flax seeds
4. Walnuts
5. Omega 9 fatty acid foods: olive oil, avocados, pecans, almonds, peanuts, cashews, sesame oil, pistachio nuts, and macadamia nuts (make sure, however, that you don't have an allergy to nuts before eating any of these foods)
6. Red pepper and cayenne pepper[163]

---

[162] Baylor College of Medicine; Proudfoot C. J., et al. Current Biology, 16. 1591 - 1605 (2006)

[163] Researchers at Wright State University report that "topical capsicum [chili pepper] is considered effective...for the temporary relief of pain from rheumatoid arthritis, osteoarthritis, and relief of neuralgias due to shingles or diabetic neuropathy... Capsicum has been approved by the Food and Drug Administration as an OTC drug for treatment of these conditions." Oral use of capsicum is not recommended due to possible liver and kidney problems.

7. Feverfew
8. Turmeric
9. White willow bark (contains salicin, which a pain blocker)[164]
10. Magnesium-rich foods (yellow vegetables)
11. Yucca[165]
12. Pineapples[166]

---

[164] Duke, PhD, James, The Green Pharmacy: In Europe, white willow bark is prescribed as an effective pain reliever for a wide spectrum of problems, from headache to arthritis.

[165] Yucca contains natural, steroidal-like saponins that are effective anti-inflammatories and anti-spasmodics known to reduce the pain associated with arthritis

[166] Bromelain, found in pineapples, has a powerful anti-inflammatory effect, which may offer pain relief with conditions such as arthritis.

Avoiding Migraines

What if you could banish migraine headaches by making changes in the foods you eat? These headaches are often painful and debilitating. Would it be worth adjusting your daily diet to avoid the pain?

In the late 1990s, Loma Linda University's School of Public Health showed that a low-fat, high-complex-carbohydrate diet can dramatically lower the frequency of migraine headaches.

The objective of the study was to reduce the fat consumption of the subjects to between twenty and thirty grams of fat per day, which was about 10 to 15 percent of total calories eaten. The results of the Loma Linda University study "demonstrated clearly a very strong connection between high dietary fat intake and migraine headache. Patients who had decreased their fat intake had significantly lowered the frequency, intensity, and duration of their migraine headaches... One of the most important contributions of the study was to identify increased levels of blood fat as the common denominator of primary headaches. These findings linked together a multitude of seemingly unrelated headache triggers, all of which cause levels of blood fat to rise. This opened the path toward a radically new treatment of headaches based on specific lifestyle modifications to reduce blood fat levels and to restore the body's natural biochemical balances necessary to prevent headaches."[167]

Diet-oriented practitioners are involved with identifying the connection between health problems and the foods people eat. This is not always easy to do, but somewhere down the line, when you can identify a problematic food or set of foods, the results of better health are well worth the effort. It takes a commitment to changing the way you eat to get to the bottom of your problem.

Some of the most important foods to eat for migraine relief are those containing magnesium—including yellow and green vegetables, such as squash and spinach. Magnesium is also found in cacao, which may be one reason why women crave chocolate around their menstrual

---

[167] Diet May Be the Key to Avoiding Painful Migraines, Nutrition Research Center online, Nov 24, 08

cycles, when the mineral is most needed for biochemical functions. Other magnesium-rich foods include nuts, almonds, artichoke hearts, avocados, sesame seeds, cashews, beans, wheat germ, legumes, seeds, meats, and certain seafoods.

Researchers at the U.S. Agricultural Research Service report, "Studies show that about half of migraine headache sufferers have a low amount of ionized magnesium in the blood, which suggests a low magnesium status. And magnesium supplementation reduces the number and duration of migraines, including menstrual migraines, in some people. The findings suggest that too little magnesium can worsen the suffering from migraine headaches."[168]

Migraines Often Have A Psychological Component

And one more important note about migraine headaches: They may be psychologically induced. While the pain and other symptoms are very real, migraine headaches can be caused by suppressing emotions such as rage. Since this rage is stored unconsciously, the migraine sufferer has no idea that it even exists or is causing headaches. The anger creates oxygen deprivation in the neck and head that may lead to a headache. Oftentimes, merely recognizing unconscious anger as a cause, and keeping your mind on emotional issues instead of the pain, will get rid of the headache. It takes some persistence to achieve success by continually thinking about this possibility until your brain gets the message. For more on this topic, read *The Divided Mind* by John Sarno, MD.

---

[168] Nielsen, Forrest H, Migraines, Sleeplessness, Heart Attacks - Magnesium?, Agricultural Research Service, United States Department of Agriculture, 2009

Borage Oil For Eczema

Skin problems involving itching, flaking, and inflammation tend to be systemic. In other words, they have to do with more than the skin itself. This is why topical ointments and creams rarely get rid of them. Diet is extremely important if you have eczema, psoriasis, Grover's Disease, or any other skin problem.

Eczema is a complicated health issue. Taking oils (like evening primrose oil) is only part of the solution. If you have eczema, you may want to go on a diet that's completely gluten-free for at least eight months, the time it takes for your digestive tract to recover from gluten's negative effects on the small intestine. Also try omitting eggs, peanuts, chocolate, dairy, and tomatoes. In addition, be aware that skin problems are frequently associated with unresolved psychological issues.

Borage Oil Decreases Itching By 90 Percent

Researchers at the University of Italy conducted a twelve-week study in 1997 that documented the dramatic effects borage oil can have on patients with atopic eczema. Of sixty patients, thirty were treated with 548 mg of GLA (gamma linolenic acid—a fatty acid found in vegetable oil) per day, while the rest received a placebo. Patients in the group receiving borage oil experienced significant reductions in all their symptoms by the end of the twelve weeks of therapy: Itching decreased about 90 percent; vesicle (small blister) formation decreased more than 40 percent; erythema (patchy redness of the skin) and oozing showed similar improvements. While positive changes in symptoms were evident during the first four weeks of treatment, the full extent of the benefits was achieved after twelve weeks. Furthermore, researchers observed that in most cases, the effects of GLA continued several weeks or months after stopping supplementation.[169]

Laboratory Findings Confirm The Benefits Of GLA Supplementation

---

[169] Artur Klimaszewski, MD, Bioriginal Publishing, October 1999; www.fatsforhealth.com/library/libitems/skin.php

Researchers in another placebo-controlled study—this time with 160 patients at six European sites—analyzed the effects of borage oil on patients with atopic eczema. The treatment group received 690 mg of GLA daily for twenty-four weeks. In patients who complied with the borage oil treatment, researchers found a significant improvement in symptoms, as compared to the placebo. Additionally, laboratory data confirmed improvements in symptoms evaluated visually and subjectively by the physician and patients. Researchers found that, in the borage oil–treatment group, the blood levels of Class E Immunoglobin, usually associated with atopic eczema, dropped dramatically.[170]

Getting The GLA You Need

Essential fatty acid researcher Artur Klimaszewski, MD, a scientist with Bioriginal Food and Science Corporation, Canada, reports, "The best source of GLA is borage (or starflower) oil, which contains up to 23 percent GLA. Evening primrose oil (8-10 percent GLA) and black currant oil (15-17 percent GLA) are other sources of GLA. Because of the higher concentration of GLA in borage, a patient may consume fewer capsules overall to achieve the required dosage. This makes borage oil the most economical source of GLA. One has to consume only 2 to 3 grams of borage oil per day to obtain an effective dosage. Studies have shown that borage oil is safe and non-toxic, even in large amounts."[171]

Dietary suggestions for skin problems include eliminating:
- Bad fats
- Artificial ingredients
- Drying agents
- Makeup that clogs pores
- Peanut butter
- Allergens in foods
- Wind, dry climate, extreme temperatures
- Harsh soaps
- Gluten-containing foods

---

[170] ibid
[171] ibid

Not Taking Acne At Face Value

The issue of acne is one on which medical doctors and natural health doctors seem to disagree, in terms of its causes and remedies. Modern medicine is inclined to treat acne as an isolated skin condition and uses chemical peels, creams, antibiotics, and other pharmaceuticals to address lesions, pimples, cysts, and blackheads. Natural healthcare doctors look at all problems of the skin as systemic. In other words, treating merely the skin is not enough because the problem really arises from the body and mind. Emotions, diet, allergies, food sensitivities, hormonal fluctuations, and stress levels all play a part in creating acne.

The cause of acne is complex in that several physiological and biochemical occurrences take place which may lead to the blockage of specific pores. This results in the build-up of materials such as sebaceous oils, cellular debris, white blood cells, and bacteria. When the pores become blocked, natural oils cannot easily exit the skin. Add to this the process of inflammation and the result is a pimple, blackhead, or cyst.

There is also often a hormonal factor adding to acne flare-ups, because sebaceous gland activity is regulated by several hormones. An imbalance in any hormonal system can contribute to acne. Since the teenage years (and puberty) mark a period of much hormonal activity, acne is more prevalent in youngsters. However, it is not uncommon to find hormonal disruptions much later down the line that contribute to adult acne, often related to female hormonal fluctuation (in women), dietary intake, etc. Also prevalent in acne cases are blood-sugar fluctuations.

Because hormonal activity, healthy skin tissue, and healthy elimination processes all may be affected by nutrition (what is consumed in the daily diet), many natural health practitioners have seen great results in treating acne when people maintain a "good" diet. This concept may be met with initial rejection by teenagers who enjoy the freedom to eat pizzas, sodas, peanut butter, and junk foods, but the choice of good nutrition becomes clear when the alternative is an out-of-control skin condition. And, you can't merely cut out a pizza once a week then expect great results. You need to be consistent and rarely, if ever, eat offensive foods.

Although it is common for dermatologists to claim that diet and nutrition have nothing to do with acne, there are thousands of doctors (and acne sufferers utilizing self-treatment) who have seen remarkable results from adhering to a good diet for an extended period of time—over the course of months. A short, one- to two-week trial on a good diet may not be quite enough time to see a significant turn around, so have patience. It takes time for your body's cells to be purged of toxins and for your organs to rebound.

For acne sufferers, even more important than giving up good-tasting but troublesome foods is eliminating "non-foods." Non-foods have either no nutritional value, contain chemicals, or have been so altered via over-processing that they fail to provide support for (and thus ultimately alter) cellular activity, as well as impair normal biochemical activity.

Give These Up To Get Rid Of Acne:

• **Altered oils**: hydrogenated and partially hydrogenated refined oils are found in refined oil/fat-based salad dressings, peanut butter, roasted nuts and seeds, potato chips, margarine, olestra, palm oil, french fries, fried foods, and mayonnaise.
Replace with: organic, unrefined coconut oil and other pure, unrefined oils (including extra virgin olive oil), salad dressings with a base of extra virgin olive oil, raw almond butter, raw nuts and seeds, corn chips, butter, baked potatoes, and other fats that naturally occur in whole foods.

• **Refined sugars**: table sugar, white sugar, brown sugar, corn sugar, corn syrup, fructose, high-fructose corn syrup, refined maple syrup, agave, and turbinado sugar. Beware of sugars in cereals (and *on* cereals, sometimes referred to as "frosted"), cola drinks, fruit drinks (that aren't 100 percent unrefined juice), and condiments like ketchup and barbecue sauce.
Replace with: stevia, honey, raw maple syrup, and products that only use stevia, honey, and raw maple syrup for sweeteners.

• **Pasteurized and homogenized dairy products**: offending milk products and processed cheeses (including "American" cheese and "cheese food") can be found in cheese pizza, ice cream, milk shakes, and cream cheese. Even soy or rice milk products may be disagreeable because they've been heated before packaging.
Replace with: raw dairy products and cheeses.

• **Other refined foods containing or processed with refined sugars, chocolate, artificial flavors/coloring and preservatives**: All of these may disrupt the hormonal system by unbalancing essential fats, vitamins, trace minerals, minerals (including calcium, magnesium, potassium, etc.), and other nutrients.

Replace with: non-refined foods with natural coloring and natural flavors, and without preservatives.

Avoid chlorine and fluoride in any form, including water for drinking, bathing, and cooking. Keep the skin washed with chemical-free soap and water. The use of topical acne creams and offensive make-up is ill-advised, though acne's cause is mostly internal, not topical.

The causes of acne have eluded doctors up to this point in time. A clean diet, finding a way to balance hormones, and applying the right type of herbs to your skin are all part of the program to eradicate this problem.

Fibroid-Fighting Foods

A diet full of seafood, including fish and seaweed, is full of iodine—an essential mineral needed by all cells, especially those of the female organs.

Iodine has long been regarded as a substance needed for the health of the thyroid gland. Unfortunately, this is as far as most healthcare practitioners go in crediting iodine for its multiplicity of uses. Just a little peek below the surface reveals a whole world of iodine-dependent functions that can make the difference between health and illness. Nearly every cell in the body needs iodine, and as of recently, several medical doctors have been studying iodine for its unique role in fighting breast and other cancers, as well as fibroids, bacterial infections, and viral illnesses.

People in the U.S. consume an average of 240 micrograms (µg) of iodine a day. In contrast, people in Japan consume more than 12 mg of iodine a day (12,000 µg), a fifty-fold greater amount.[172]

According to iodine expert David Brownstein, MD, besides providing thyroid health, iodine has other functions "that require more study. It removes toxic chemicals—fluoride, bromide, lead, aluminum, mercury—and biological toxins, suppresses auto-immunity, strengthens the T-cell adaptive immune system, and protects against abnormal growth of bacteria in the stomach."[173] Certain substances called halides—like fluoride, chloride, and bromide (used in baking)—interfere with your body's ability to use iodine and may lead to health problems. The problem is that halides compete with (and win against) iodine for receptor sites in cells. This is one of many arguments against fluoridating the water supply—fluoride will crowd out iodine so your cells will be deprived of this life-supporting nutrient.

Dr. Brownstein's initial research into iodine showed that out of 500 patients, nearly 95 percent were iodine deficient.

---

[172] Miller, Jr., M.D., Donald W., Extrathyroidal Benefits of Iodine , Journal of American Physicians and Surgeons Volume 11 Number 4 Winter 2006
[173] Brownstein, MD, David, Clinical Experience with Inorganic Non-radioactive Iodine/Iodide

Regarding fibrocystic breast disease, alternative medicine advocate Jonathan Wright, MD, stated:

In the 1970s, I learned from pioneering trace element researcher, Dr. John Myers, that iodine...would eliminate even the most severe cases of fibrocystic breast disease. For the full details of this treatment....In 'medium' to 'minor' cases, 6 to 8 drops of SSKI [potassium iodide] taken in a few ounces of water daily will frequently reduce fibrocystic breast disease to insignificance within three to six months. Please do not do this without monitoring your thyroid function...One of our daughters and at least thirty other women I've worked with in nearly 30 years have helped ovarian cysts disappear within two to three months with the same quantity of SSKI. Again, make sure to monitor your thyroid function![174]

Many times we'll hear of people who say they are allergic to iodine. Is this really possible if iodine is an absolute necessity for cellular function throughout our bodies? Dr. Wright notes, "The type of so-called 'iodine allergy' that can interfere with breathing and occasionally sends us to the emergency room is usually not allergy to iodine or iodine molecules, but instead to much larger, possibly iodine-containing molecules found in lobster, crab, clams and other 'shellfish.' These molecules are not present in SSKI or iodine. However, if there's any suspicion at all of iodine allergy, it's best not to swallow any without testing for allergy or sensitivity... Iodine allergy is a possibility, although in nearly 30 years of medical practice I've seen it only a few times. Usually, it causes a red, bumpy skin rash, which goes away after SSKI or other iodine is discontinued. Topical (applied to the skin surface) iodine allergy is almost never a serious emergency."[175]

More On The Iodine-Allergy Confusion
Iodine may be used topically for many health concerns, including for toenail fungus, yeast infections, warts, moles, skin keratoses, and infections.

Physician, researcher, and author David Derry, MD, writes, "There has been no significant clinical research on iodine therapy or use for 40 years...I feel it is important for research to be directed at this

---

[174] Wright, MD, Jonathan, "One mineral can help a myriad of conditions from atherosclerosis to COPD to zits, tahoma-clinic.com/iodide.shtml, 2008
[175] ibid

potentially significant area of medical treatment. It is worth noting the greatest part of significant research with iodine was done before the Medline search facilities were available. Of course, since large doses of iodine are tolerated intravenously without side effects, it has yet to be explored what help this may have for many cancer patients or even other diseases."[176]

The best way to get iodine into your cells is to eat lots and lots of seafood. But make certain you first do a little research online to determine which fish has the lowest traces of unsafe metals such as mercury.

---

[176] Dr. David Derry Answers Reader Questions Brought to you by Mary Shomon, Your Thyroid Guide; 2009; http://thyroid.about.com/library/derry/bl2a.htm

Super Foods For Sinus Problems

If you have sinus problems, a clean lifestyle and a diet full of Super Foods may be the solution.

The sinuses are cavities found within the head, face, and nose. When any of these areas become inflamed, the pain and suffering can become unbearable. Milder forms of sinus problems may include stuffy or runny nose, sniffling, mucous drip, bad breath, slight breathing difficulties, coughing, foggy thinking, sneezing, and altered speaking patterns (talking through your nose or talking with a blocked nose, for example).

What causes sinus problems? There is no single answer. Some people are more sensitive than others in this area and may be affected by strong perfumes, garbage or paint fumes, smoke (cigarette, fireplace, or other kinds), traffic exhaust, dust, pet dander and fur, fatty foods, and dairy products. Whatever causes an overabundance of mucous can cause sinus headaches or other such symptoms. If you think you're affected by changes in the weather, you should look into other possible causes; humidity may be more of a trigger than an actual cause.

There has been speculation that some sinus problems may be caused by food intolerance, including problems with gluten. Avoiding gluten in all foods may be necessary if no other remedies seem to work. Gluten avoidance must be complete and practiced for a period of no less than eight months to see if it is at the root of your sinus problems.

If your sinuses give you trouble, try your best to avoid the following for at least a few weeks and see how you feel:

* Eggs
* Milk, cream, margarine, cream cheese, cheese, and other dairy products
* Chocolate
* All strong chemical odors (perfumes, glues, etc.)
* Dust and pollution
* Plant pollen (try to stay indoors if plants are in bloom)
* Drugs (check side effects with your doctor or the PDR)
* Cigarette smoke and environmental smoke (fireplaces, forest fires, etc.)

- Artificial ingredients in foods (chemicals, trans-fats, etc.); switch to **ORGANIC** foods
- Fried foods and bad oils (trans-fats, canola, cooked oils, etc.)
- Fatty foods (fatty meats, creamy foods, sauces, gravies, etc.)
- Refined sugars (soft drinks, powdered drinks, syrups, desserts, etc.)
- All drinks except organic green tea, decaffeinated tea, and water
- Processed foods (foods in packages—except for organic grains and oatmeal—including chips, boxed cereals, canned foods, crackers, and junk foods)

Doctors who specialize in sinus conditions also recommend avoiding histamine foods. Allergists Jeffrey Tulin-Silver, MD, and Suchetha Kinhal, MD, report:

Histamine is a vasoactive amine which causes dilatation of the blood vessels (flushing, rash, itching) and increased mucus production (runny nose, productive cough), and bronchoconstriction (wheezing, cough). Because histamine is contained in almost all body tissues, especially the lungs, nose, sinuses, skin, intestinal mucosa and certain blood cells (mast cells, basophils), it is able to cause a wide variety of symptoms...

There are many foods that contain histamine or cause the body to release histamine when ingested. These types of reactions are food intolerances, and are different from food allergy in that the immune system is not involved in the reaction. The symptoms, however, can be the same as a food allergy. Foods that contain the chemical *tyramine* can trigger headaches. Foods that may have large amounts of tyramine include: fish, chocolate, alcoholic beverages, cheese, soy sauce, sauerkraut and processed meat. Fermented foods may cause allergy symptoms because they are either rich in histamine or because yeast or mold is involved in the fermentation process.[177]

Sinus Infections—Antibiotics Are Not Always The Answer

---

[177] Tulin-Silver, MD, and Suchetha Kinhal, MD, Foods that contain histamine or cause the body to release histamine, including fermented foods, Michigan Allergy, Sinus & Asthma Specialists, michiganfoodallergy.net, West Bloomfield, MI, 2009

Health researcher Kimberley Beauchamp, ND, explains, "Although the majority of sinus infections are not caused by bacteria, antibiotics (which kill only bacteria) are the most commonly prescribed drug treatment. [An] important possibility is that many patients have self-limited disease that will resolve regardless of treatment."[178] In other words, even though the antibiotics appear to have cleared up the infection, it might have happened just as quickly with no treatment at all. There are concerns about the overuse of antibiotics and the resultant problems, including drug resistance and increasingly virulent bacteria.

Manual Treatment

Sometimes sinus pressure may be relieved by vigorously massaging facial sinuses, receiving acupuncture treatment, drinking a couple cups of strong organic coffee, applying ice packs to the area, rigorously exercising, neck massage, sleep, or practicing certain breathing exercises.

Or you can flush out your sinuses. Using a neti pot or bulb syringe with pure water to cleanse the nasal passages and sinuses is highly effective for treating both acute and chronic sinusitis. It can also be helpful (especially for chronic sinusitis) to identify and treat food allergies and intolerances.[179]

Super Foods For Sinuses

Some of the more useful Super Foods for relieving sinus problems include garlic, broccoli, Echinacea, Pau d'arco, onions, fish oils, evening primrose oil, flax seed oil, and, when treating extreme sinus headaches, a couple of cups of hot organic coffee, if you can tolerate it. Sinus problems are mostly the effect of long-term dietary imbalances and are not easily corrected with supplements or a quick fix. If you suffer from chronic sinus conditions, it's best to completely clean up your diet and avoid dairy, most oils, and any other food that causes congestion. By simplifying your diet and eating the Super Foods discussed in this book, you will, by trial and error, realize which foods most aggravate your condition.

At one point, doctors said that eating spicy foods would help to clear sinuses. But recent research shows otherwise. Hot foods such as

---

[178] Beauchamp, ND, Kimberly, "Sinus Infections — Antibiotics Not Always the Answer," Healthnotes Newswire; April 5, 2007
[179] Arch Otolaryngol Head Neck Surg 2007;133:260–5

peppers, wasabi, horseradish, and others make your nose run at first, giving the false impression that they're working magic. However, doctors at Oakland's Kaiser Permanente Medical Center say that wasabi and other spicy foods are good only for temporary symptom relief, causing a runny nose and sinuses that seem to be draining. But in fact, these foods make things worse for your sinuses. All that's happening is that *allylisothiocyanate*—the pungent ingredient found in wasabi, horseradish, and mustard—is causing a burning sensation in the nose, which activates a certain muscle to allow for more air to enter the sinuses. Receptors within the nose then tell your brain that you're breathing easier. Unfortunately, your nose is only fooling your brain. Thus, say researchers, eating spicy foods ultimately produces greater nasal congestion and increased mucus production.[180]

---

[180] Cameron David S and Raul M Cruz, Department of Head and Neck Surgery at Kaiser Permanente Medical Center, Oakland, California, 2004

Mouth Sores Driving You Crazy?

Mouth sores are more than just a pain. They keep you from eating, kissing, brushing your teeth, chewing, and even smiling. Researchers are very conflicted over what causes them, but the authors of this book have a few theories of their own as to some nutritional correlations.

Many people deal with the bane of sores appearing from time to time inside their lips or cheeks. Such sores often appear as a whitish spot, about the size of a pencil eraser. It's painful to the touch and doesn't seem to want to go away. Although the sore—more aptly described as an ulceration—is visible, it's only a sign that there's a problem inside your body.

If You Develop Mouth Sores, You May Want To Follow These Suggestions:

1. Do not eat any black pepper, spicy peppers, or hot spices
2. Take 2000μ of natural vitamin D3 every day for ten days (available at most health food stores)
3. Take a calcium-magnesium supplement
4. Eat a lot of vitamin C foods, like lemons, oranges, and berries (Camu-Camu is a super vitamin C food from the Amazon that can be found in supplement form)
5. Avoid sugar and sugar-containing foods until the sore goes away
6. Avoid all hard, crispy, sharp foods, such as pretzels, potato chips, breadsticks, and nuts
7. Avoid all salty foods
8. Avoid chocolate
9. Avoid gluten (cold sores are often associated with gluten intolerance as well)
10. Go on a three-day vegetable juice fast using a wide variety of vegetables each serving

Nutritional deficiencies leading to mouth sores include a lack of foods that contain minerals (mainly green vegetable foods)— especially calcium, a lack of vitamin C foods, an unbalanced diet, hard-to-tolerate foods (including pepper, salt, spices, etc.), and even gluten intolerance (for many people). It is also common for sores on, in, and around the mouth to be associated with emotional stress and anger.

Feeding The Mind And Emotions

Emotional and mental health have more to do with than just the way you look at things. You have to feed your brain special nutrients to fuel psychological processes. If your diet is deficient in certain building blocks, your brain will not be able to make neurotransmitters, the chemicals responsible for sending nerve impulses from cell to cell. If you don't have enough neurotransmitters, the result may be neurological and mental disorders. This can mean anything from not being able to think clearly to experiencing excessive worry, depression, and so forth.

Chemicals that are used by your body to make neurotransmitters include aspartic acid—found in peanuts, potatoes, eggs, and grains; choline—found in eggs, liver, and soybeans; glutamic acid—found in flour and potatoes; phenylalanine (used to make dopamine)—found in beets, soybeans, almonds, eggs, meat, and grains; tryptophan (used to make serotonin)—found in eggs, meat, skim milk, bananas, yogurt, milk, and cheese; and tyrosine (used to make *norepinephrine*)—found in milk, meat, fish, and legumes.[181]

What does any of this have to do with your being happy, emotionally, and mentally balanced? This is a loaded question because there are so many factors, chemically speaking, that affect your brain and, in turn, emotion and thought processes. To give you an idea, these factors include hormones, oxygen, blood sugar, genetics, exercise, patterned responses to stress and other problems, and worldview (the way you tend to look at things), as well as the effects of sugars and artificial ingredients, drugs, excitotoxins, and other poisons. However, there are a few nutrients that always benefit your brain, including vitamin B complex in foods, as well as good fats, minerals, and proteins.

Thiamine (vitamin B1)—in legumes, grains, and some seeds— is needed for maintaining your energy supplies and coordinating the activity of nerves and muscles. A deficiency can lead to weakness, irritability, and depression. Folate (vitamin B9)—found in leafy greens,

---

[181] Chudler, PhD, Eric, University of Washington Engineered Biomaterials in Seattle, Washington, faculty.washington.edu/chudler/nutr.html

legumes, and fortified grains—is essential for supporting red blood cell production, helping prevent homocysteine build-up in your blood and allowing nerves to function properly. Folate deficiency can result in depression, apathy, fatigue, poor sleep, and poor concentration.

Scientists discovered that the omega-3 fats in cod liver oil fight depression,[182] as do folate and vitamin B12 in foods.[183] Meats such as turkey, tuna, and chicken are rich in an amino acid called tyrosine, which helps to raise levels of dopamine and norepinephrine chemicals in the brain, helping you to feel more alert and focused.[184] If you have a child with attention deficit disorder (ADD), consider getting all artificial ingredients out of his or her diet.[185]

One of the most treasured foods for elevating the mood is chocolate. Researchers in Wales report, "There have been a series of suggestions that chocolate's mood elevating properties reflect 'drug-like' constituents including anandamines, caffeine, phenylethylamine and magnesium. However, the levels of these substances are so low as to preclude such influences. As all palatable foods stimulate endorphin release in the brain this is the most likely mechanism to account for the elevation of mood."[186]

University of Illinois nutritionist Gillian Goodfriend notes, "Remember, vitamins and minerals from food are much more readily and efficiently absorbed in the body than those obtained from supplements. By eating a wide variety of foods—including lean proteins, whole grains, fruits, vegetables, healthy fats, and low-fat dairy products—you are bound to obtain the nutrients needed to support a healthy body and mind."[187]

Vitamin B-containing foods that are good for your mind and emotions include yeast, rice bran extract, defatted wheat germ, sprouted barley malt, astragalus, oat bran, beet root, liver, figs, and sunflower seeds. And if you're under stress (who isn't these days?), you'll burn off more vitamin B complex; so you always have to have a fresh supply of these foods. Good fats for your brain are found in cod liver oil, fish oils, olive oil, coconut butter, evening primrose oil, and borage oil.

---

[182] J Affect Disord. 2007 Aug;101(1-3):245-9. Epub 2006 Dec 19

[183] J Psychopharmacol. 2005 Jan;19(1):59-65

[184] Chakraburtty, MD, Amal, Diet for Depression, webmd.com Nov 08

[185] Lancet. 2007 Nov 3;370(9598):1560-7

[186] The Effects of Nutrients on Mood, Public Health Nutr. 1999 Sep;2(3A):403-9

[187] Food and Your Mood: Nutrition and Mental Health, ncpad.org/nutrition/fact_sheet.php?sheet=670, USDA, mypyramid.gov, Jan 08

Especially bad for your brain are mercury (avoid predator fish as well as too much tuna, because they are notably high in toxic metals), MSG, any artificial ingredients,[188] food dyes and other chemicals, and refined sugars. In addition, more and more people are claiming that gluten foods are causing mental and emotional problems. Cutting all gluten out of the diet has made a world of difference for thousands of people.

---

[188] "Since its 1981 approval, the FDA has published a list of 92 symptoms of aspartame poisoning, which includes headaches, vision loss including blindness, seizures, neurological problems, cardiovascular problems and death. The FDA admits adverse reactions to aspartame comprise about 80 percent of consumer complaints it receives each year," yet the political power of the makers of this artificial ingredient outweighs public health, thanks in large part to Donald Rumsfeld: "Three years after Donald Rumsfeld became CEO of Searle, aspartame was approved for use in dry goods. To find out how he accomplished this feat, click into the new movie, "Sweet Misery: A Poisoned World" and hear the words of renowned Washington Consumer Attorney James Turner as he speaks about President Reagan's Executive Order: http://www.soundandfury.tv/pages/Rumsfeld2.html; organicconsumers.org/toxic/aspartame.cfm, dorway.com

Wheat Germ Calms Your Nerves

In a symposium held in London 1939, Dr. Vogt-Moeller, a researcher who was ahead of his time, proclaimed, "Finally, let it be kept in mind that wheat germ oil, which so far has been the preparation most commonly employed for therapeutic trials, may contain many biologically active substances other than Vitamin E...."[189]

Essentially, he was saying what many before and after him have claimed —that foods contain much more than just the vitamins or minerals that scientists show to have health benefits. Vogt-Moeller insisted that various reports on vitamin E's influence on neuromuscular disorders are confusing because vitamin E was used in some experiments, while wheat germ oil was used in others. It has been shown previously that wheat germ oil contains factors other than vitamin E.[190]

Vogt-Moeller created an experiment involving ninety dogs affected by distemper. All dogs (including the controls) were placed on a balanced diet with a supplementary vitamin B-complex preparation. Before instituting treatment, he waited until all dogs had developed the initial symptoms of the disease, prior to developing the next stage of neuromuscular disturbances.

Thirty dogs were injected daily with 10 mg of alpha tocopherol (vitamin E). Thirty dogs were injected daily with 5cc of wheat germ oil, which contained 10mg of alpha tocopherol. And, of course, the remaining thirty dogs were given nothing at all.

In the final analysis, Vogt-Moeller offered that wheat germ oil contains a factor other than vitamin E that exerts a beneficial effect.191 The lesson we get from his work is that although scientists may identify vitamins within foods, the vitamins alone are not all we need to fulfill our nutritional requirements.

---

[189] Levin, MA, Ezra, "Vitamin E vs. Wheat Germ Oil," American Journal of Digestive Diseases, Vol 12, No 1, p. 20, Monticello, IL, 1944
[190] Martin, G. J. : J. Nutrition, 13:679; 1937
[191] American Journal of Digestive Diseases, Vol. 12, no.1, Jan, 1945. pages 20-21

Wheat germ oil is an excellent source of vitamin E, a nutrient needed for health of the heart, skin, nervous system, hormones, etc., but it also contains other factors in the plant oil that support a great number of systems in the body.

Wheat germ oil is extracted from the germ of the wheat kernel and has the highest vitamin E content of any food that has not undergone prior preparation or vitamin fortification. Wheat germ oil contains beneficial fatty acids including linoleic acid (omega 6), palmitic acid, oleic acid, and linoleic acid (omega-3). It also contains vitamin K, and choline.[192] Wheat germ's octacosanol increases athletic performance and helps lower cholesterol levels.[193]

If you take wheat germ oil, make sure that it's cold-pressed, organic, and not processed with the use of hexane (a common toxic chemical used by many supplement companies).

---

[192] Nutrition facts on wheat germ oil, http://www.nutritiondata.com/facts/fats-and-oils/505/2

[193] Mitmesser, Susan H., "Octacosanol and Wheat Germ Oil", Sports Nutrition, Fats and Proteins, CRC Press, University of Nebraska, 2007

Super Foods To Lighten Depression

When people say they are depressed, they could mean that they're experiencing anything from normal occasional bouts of sadness to something much more severe.

In a given year, approximately 18.8 million American adults, or about 9.5 percent of the U.S. population aged eighteen and older, have a depressive disorder. Nearly twice as many women (12 percent) as men (6.6 percent) are affected by one each year. These figures translate to 12.4 million women and 6.4 million men in the United States alone. Not only that, but people born in recent decades may be acquiring depressive disorders earlier in life than those before them. Depressive disorders often co-occur with anxiety disorders and substance abuse.

No matter how great one's depressive state, there are Super Foods that can help. This is because the brain and emotions respond to proper nutrition.

Depression has long been deferred to the field of psychology for treatment, yet recent scientific findings indicate that insufficient nutritional (i.e., biochemical) support may be at the root of many debilitating episodes. Leading the list of needed nutrients that your mind and emotions need for emotional support is vitamin B complex. Research has suggested a link between depression and low blood levels of folate, a B vitamin, and a new study from the Friedman School of Nutrition at Tufts University strengthens the association. Investigators looked at folate concentrations in about 3,000 people and found deficiencies that correlated with mental and emotional problems.[194] This makes sense, as vitamin B complex feeds the nervous system and the brain.

B vitamins feed and regulate brain chemistry. Vitamin B complex is used to create the neurotransmitters known as serotonin and catecholamines (adrenaline and norepinephrine). Plus, vitamin B complex is essential for the production of *S-adenosylme-thionine*, a chemical with antidepressant properties.

---

[194] Health & Nutrition Letter, B Vitamin May Help Ease Depression, Tufts University, August 2003

Dr. James Meschino, in his article on vitamin B and memory in senior citizens, wrote:

> Vitamin B12 deficiency may also result in de-insulation of nerve fibers (demyelination), which produces a constellation of neurological symptoms. Vitamin B6 is a cofactor in the production of other brain chemicals (neurotransmitters), including dopamine, norepinephrine, serotonin, GABA, and taurine...Taken together, the body of evidence continues to support the contention that B vitamin nutritional status is crucial to the development and preservation of mental capacities throughout one's lifetime.

The sad reality is that many...members of society have poor dietary intake and nutritional status of various B vitamins (vitamin B6, folic acid, etc.). By all counts, it appears that health practitioners should encourage patients to pay attention to foods that are rich sources of these, and to continue to emphasize the multitude of benefits available from the daily use of a well-formulated multiple vitamin and mineral supplement.[195]

Unfortunately, most people try taking isolated vitamin B complex supplements (instead of the actual vitamin B foods) and see little or no improvement in their condition. Many times their vitamin pills make them sick. This is because such vitamin pills are not foods, but rather chemicals and are lacking the synergists (helper nutrients) found in vitamin B-containing natural, whole foods. If you're looking for a supplemental source of B vitamins, it is best to use a non-sterilized, whole-food formula product that includes a variety of vitamin B–containing foods—not one that's been infused with isolated vitamins or altered through heating or any other unnatural means.

Emotional Problems—Not So Simple To Define
As with every health condition, there may be several causes for emotional problems. Many, though, are created or made worse by a deficiency of the vitamin B complex. Such problems include faulty neurotransmission, brain chemical imbalances, and hormonal dysfunction (which may require eating specific foods and herbs known to support endocrine/glandular health).

---

[195] B Vitamins May Hold Key to Better Memory, Cognitive Function in Seniors, James Meschino, DC, MS, http://www.chiroweb.com/archives/20/22/11.html

Other causes of depression may be mostly psychological in origin and require counseling or other psychological treatment. Yet, because the body and mind are intricately connected, finding food sources of B vitamins and other pertinent nutrients is helpful as part of a well-rounded approach to depression.

Fruits & Berries Bolster Carotid Arteries

Fruits and berries are good for your cardiovascular system. In early 2009, the journal *Nutrition, Metabolism and Cardiovascular Diseases*, reported that researchers from Ulleval University Hospital in Norway showed a diet high in fruit and berries were associated with less thickening of the carotid artery.[196]

The carotid artery is the main blood vessel that leads from the heart up through the neck and is one of the most popular sites for plaque build-up and blockages. Fortunately, the nutritional content of fruits and berries may be the best way to avoid surgeries to remove plaque and repair blood vessels. As these foods eliminate plaque, more blood can flow from the head and into the brain, as well as throughout every part of the body, reducing heart attacks, stroke, poor circulation, and pain.

Fruits and berries contain vitamin C, a nutrient that won a great deal of popularity when researcher Linus Pauling first fought to popularize the notion that the common cold can be treated with megadoses. However, ascorbic acid is NOT THE BEST source of vitamin C because it's artificial and does not contain other important nutrients that are found in nature's fruits and berries. The BEST SOURCE of vitamin C is from real, natural, and *whole* foods—not pills.

If you can eat a daily helping lemons, limes, oranges, apples, and other fruits, as well as berries, you're getting a great source of vitamin C. If you need an additional boost, Camu-Camu is a rainforest fruit that has the highest known concentrated source of vitamin C.

What's more, it's not just your heart, but all the cells in your body that require vitamin C—from bones to gums and from arteries to skin.[197] So make sure your diet is supplying enough to keep you in the pink.

---

[196] Daniells, Stephen, "Vitamin C-rich foods may boost artery health, nutraingredients.com,Feb-2009, and Nutrition, Metabolism and Cardiovascular Diseases, Volume 19, Issue 1, Pages 8-14
[197] ibid

Heart Support from Three Ancient Foods

Heart problems abound in America, manifesting in a variety of ways—atherosclerosis, chest pains, fibrillation, high blood pressure, blocked arteries, deteriorated valves, poor circulation, etc. Dean Ornish, MD, clinical professor of medicine at the University of California–San Francisco, tells us that almost all heart diseases can be cured and avoided by diet and lifestyle changes alone, without medications or surgery. While this doesn't necessarily make bypass surgeons happy and rich, it should be great news to the rest of us.

With all the modern medical approaches to heart disease, natural healthcare still endorses three traditional foods that continue to support the entire cardiovascular system. Medical research continues to show that the fantastic properties of grapes, hawthorn berries, and green tea—three ancient foods—are effective in cardiovascular prevention and healing.

One active ingredient of note in grapes is in a class called *Oligomeric proanthocyanidins* (OPC). Dietitian Marilyn Sterling writes, "Proanthocyanidins deserve their stellar reputation as antioxidants that quench free radicals and potentiate other antioxidants. A recent mouse study by Debasis Bagchi, Ph.D., and colleagues at the Creighton University School of Pharmacy in Omaha, Nebraska, also found that their grape seed extract protected tissue from oxidation better than the antioxidant vitamins C and E or beta-carotene."[198]

According to animal studies, OPCs appear to inhibit several factors contributing to atherosclerosis. Proanthocyanidins may help explain what has been termed the "French Paradox"—why low coronary heart disease rates exist in French provinces despite diets filled with high-fat foods and ample red wine. Red wine could be considered an alcohol tincture of several potent flavonoids, including

---

[198] Sterling, RD, Marilyn, Proanthocyanidin Power, Pine bark and grape seed contain the flavonoids OPCs, which offer antioxidant protection against heart disease and cancer, New Hope Media, Nutrition Science News, Jun 00

proanthocyanidins from grape seeds (see the previous chapters on Grapes and Grape Seeds for more information).

Proanthocyanidins also play a role in the stabilization of collagen and maintenance of elastin in connective tissue. So if you have sagging skin, wrinkles, leaking blood vessels, plaque build-up in your arteries, or cellulite, or if you are aging prematurely, grape seed extract and green tea may be foods you'll want to add to your Super Food diet.

Lastly, we have hawthorn berries on our list of Super Foods promoting heart health. Varro Tyler, PhD, dean and professor emeritis of pharmaconosy at Purdue University, seconds the motion that hawthorn's benefit to heart health lies in its OPCs. But she explains that other compounds within the fruit dilate blood vessels of the coronary arteries, which is why it has enjoyed a tradition of treating angina (heart pains).[199]

Note of caution: Due to hawthorn's strength, it's not advisable to use this plant food without direction from a qualified health care practitioner.

---

[199] Duke, PhD, James, The Green Pharmacy, p. 44-45

Biotin Foods For Cellular Health

Have you ever heard of biotin? It's an important B vitamin that's widely distributed in a variety of foods, but most often at low concentrations. Estimates are that the typical U.S. diet provides roughly 40 mcg a day of it. There are only a couple of foods containing biotin in large amounts, including royal jelly and brewer's yeast. Though in less concentration, the best natural sources of biotin in human nutrition are Swiss chard, tomatoes, romaine lettuce, and carrots. Other great sources include eggs, goat's milk, cow's milk, halibut, onions, cabbage, cucumber, cauliflower, raspberries, strawberries, oats, almonds, and walnuts.

Biotin is necessary for the growth of cells, the production of fatty acids, the metabolism of fats and amino acids, and the maintenance of a steady blood sugar level. It plays a role in the citric acid cycle, the process by which biochemical energy is generated during aerobic respiration. Biotin is often recommended for strengthening hair and nails and so is found in many cosmetic and health products.

Biotin deficiency is relatively rare and mild, and can be addressed with supplementation. Such a deficiency can be caused by the excessive consumption of raw egg whites, which contain high levels of the protein *avidin* that binds strongly with biotin. Avidin is deactivated by cooking, leaving the biotin intact.

Signs Of Biotin Deficiency
In general, appetite and growth are decreased when you're deficient in biotin, and many people experience dermatologic (skin) symptoms—including dermatitis, alopecia (hair loss), and achromotrichia (absence or loss of pigment in the hair), perosis (a shortening and thickening of bones), as well as liver problems (Fatty Liver and Kidney Syndrome).

Food Compounds That Kill Lab Cancer Cells

Strawberries, grapes, blueberries, and some familiar seasonings (like rosemary) contain compounds that can—at least in the laboratory—kill cells of childhood leukemia. Nutrition-focused research conducted by molecular biologist Susan J. Zunino of the Agricultural Research Service (ARS), Western Human Nutrition Research Center (WHNRC), Davis, California, may have the answer to exactly how these powerful plant chemicals fight acute lymphoblastic leukemia.

Zunino's newer studies build upon her 2006 findings about the chemical ability of carnosol, from rosemary; curcumin, from turmeric; resveratrol, from grapes; and ellagic acid, kaempferol, and quercetin, from strawberries to kill the leukemia cells. For her model, she worked with laboratory cultures of both healthy human blood cells and cancerous human blood cells.

Zunino's work gained the attention of not only cancer researchers, but nutrition scientists who explore the health benefits of natural compounds in the world's fruits, vegetables, herbs, and spices. For the most part, scientists don't yet have all the details about how plant chemicals (phytochemicals) bolster healthy cells and battle harmful ones. According to Zunino, this holds true even for better-known phytochemicals, such as the resveratrol in grapes, blueberries, bilberries, and some other fruits.

Her investigations provide some new clues about how phytochemicals attack cancer cells. For example, she found that phytochemicals interfere with the orderly operations of cancer cells' mitochondria—the miniature energy-producing power plants inside the cells. When mitochondria in cancer cells were exposed to both resveratrol and the other phytochemicals that Zunino tested, they couldn't function properly.[200] By starving cancer cells of their energy, scientists are beginning to find ways of killing them without the use of radiation and chemotherapy. But it would be wiser to merely eat plenty of nutritious foods so you don't develop cancer in the first place.

---

[200] Wood, Marcia, Agricultural Research, US Department of Agriculture, March 4, 2008

No More Confusion About Blood Sugar

The topic of blood sugar can be confusing with phrases like "too high," "too low," "out of balance," "insulin levels," "hypoglycemia," "diabetes," and so forth. What do you need to know to stay healthy? Ideally, we should all be eating a good diet consisting mostly of fruits, vegetables, nuts, seeds, berries, good grains, and a little organic meat. But most of us don't, so this is where the problem begins—even if you may be genetically predisposed to the aforementioned conditions.

Blood sugar metabolism is not a simple subject, but we'll give you the simplest version possible of what's going on in the process. When you eat sugar, your cells use it for energy and the production of fat, among other things. After you eat it, it enters your bloodstream and a hormone in your pancreas has the job of taking the sugar out of the blood and putting it into your cells. That hormone is called insulin.

So what goes wrong? When your pancreas has to work too hard, it gets worn out. Most people eat far too much sugar—about 140 pounds a year per average American! With this overabundance of sugar entering your body, you can imagine how the pancreas can become overworked and how the hormones get stressed out from having to process such a large load. If your pancreas can no longer provide enough insulin, you end up with too much sugar in your blood, which is dangerous. The problem, when chronic, is called diabetes.

On the other hand, when you don't have enough sugar in your body, you can develop hypoglycemia, which means "low blood sugar."

If you eat more glucose (sugar) than your body needs at the time, your body stores the extra glucose in your liver and muscles in a form called glycogen. Your body can use glycogen for energy between meals. Extra glucose can also be changed to fat and stored in your fat cells to be used for energy.

Doctors at the National Institutes of Health tell us, "When blood glucose begins to fall, *glucagons*—hormones made by the pancreas—tell your liver to break down glycogen and release more sugar into the bloodstream. Blood sugar then rises back to a normal level. In some people with diabetes, this glucagon response to hypoglycemia does not work normally and other hormones such as *epinephrine*, also called *adrenaline*, may be used to raise the blood

145

glucose level. But with diabetes treated with insulin or pills that increase insulin production, glucose levels can't easily return to the normal range."

Hypoglycemia can come on suddenly with symptoms such as dizziness, blackouts, fainting (or near-fainting), sweating, nervousness, difficulty speaking or focusing, confusion, anxiety, and so forth. It is usually mild and can be treated quickly and easily by eating or drinking a small amount of a glucose-rich substance, like fruit juice. But if chronic hypoglycemia is not addressed, you can pass out; and severe cases can lead to seizures, a coma, and even death. In adults and children older than age ten, hypoglycemia is uncommon, except as a side effect of diabetes treatment.[201]

Low blood sugar problems are very much a common occurrence with today's simple sugar diets. You eat ice cream and cookies, and then are loaded with sugar that's moved into your cells quickly, and you end up without enough sugar to take another step. In more graphic terms, you think you need "a sugar fix." This is bad news because you're setting yourself up for a dangerous cycle of high and low blood sugar, taxing your hormones, liver, and pancreas—not to mention other organs and glands that are affected. Hypoglycemia can also result, however, from medications or diseases, hormone or enzyme deficiencies, or tumors.

This is all just another solid reason to avoid eating sugary foods that have no redeeming nutritional value.

At the other end of the spectrum from hypoglycemia is diabetes. Nutrition researcher Dr. Maureen Williams, writes, "People with diabetes have high blood sugar levels because their cells don't respond to insulin, the hormone that signals when glucose (the form sugar takes in the blood) needs to be stored. Over time, the extra glucose in the blood damages tissues. Eating a high-fiber, low-sugar diet and exercising are important ways to keep blood glucose levels normal. Oral medications are also often used to reduce blood glucose levels, and in some cases insulin injections are necessary."[202]

Foods And Herbs That Help

---

[201] "Hypoglycemia," National Institute of Diabetes and Digestive and Kidney Diseases, National Institues of Health, Bethesda, MD, 2009
[202] Williams, ND, Maureen, Cinnamon Lowers High Blood Sugar, 2006-08-18 - healthnotes Newswire, 06

Because eating sugar is so often associated with the formation of fat, many of the foods and herbs involved in balancing blood sugar are also helpful in weight loss.

There are certainly a few good foods and herbs that support your pancreas, liver, and other systems that process sugars from foods you eat. One of special note that few people know about is an ancient Indian herb called *gymnema* (jim-nee-ma) *sylvestre* and is used in Ayurvedic (traditional Indian) medicine. We'll refer to the herb as gymnema, for short.

Practitioners of Ayurveda first used gymnema to treat diabetes almost 2,000 years ago. In the 1920s, preliminary scientific studies showed some evidence that gymnema leaves can reduce blood sugar levels, but nothing much came of this observation for decades. Research in India picked up again in the 1980s and 1990s, leading to the publication of promising studies in people.[203] The leaves (and sometimes stems) of this woody, vine-like plant are used medicinally in the treatments of diabetes, hyperglycemia, and dyslipidemia.[204]

University of Michigan Health Systems researchers tell us that gymnema leaves raise insulin levels. This may be due to regeneration of the cells in the pancreas that secrete insulin, or by increasing the flow of insulin from these cells. Animal research shows that gymnema can reduce sugar absorption from the intestine, help move glucose out of the blood and into cells, and prevent adrenal hormones from stimulating the liver to produce extra sugar. Extracts of gymnema leaves can lower serum cholesterol and trigylcerides and prevent weight gain. When placed directly on the tongue, gurmarin, another constituent of the leaves, and gymnemic acid have been shown to block the ability in humans to taste sweets.[205]

All You Need To Know

[203] "Gymnema," rev by EBSCO Complementary and Alternative Medicine (CAM) Review Board, Richard Glickman-Simon, MD, Jeffrey S. Geller, MD, et al., Sep 09; healthlibrary.epnet.com/GetContent.aspx?token=e0498803-7f62-4563-8d47-5fe33da65dd4&chunkiid=21774

[204] Pierce A. Gymnema Monograph. Practical guide to natural medicine. New York: Stonesong Press Book; 1999. p. 324-26, as cited by Oksana Federenko Reviewed 5/12/03 Susan Paulsen Pharm D, University of Colorado Denver, uchsc.edu/sop/pharmd/6.Experiential_Programs/-downloads/gymnema.pdf; 2008

[205] "Gymnema," University of Michigan Health System, Healthwise Knowledgebase, Ann Arbor, MI, 07

Scientific studies show that gymnema contains several substances that can lower blood sugar and lipid levels, increase the enzyme activity responsible for using and processing sugars, and reduce cravings for sweets.[206] Like almost every herb, be sure to look into how much you should be taking, as there is a propensity for gymnema to cause health problems if taken in large dosages. One way to avoid trouble here is to be guided by a qualified nutritional healthcare practitioner.

Cinnamon Is Another Blood-Sugar-Lowering Gem
Cinnamon is a spice that most people eat just because they like the taste. However, it shows great promise in ironing out blood sugar imbalances as well. In a study conducted at Malmo University Hospital in Sweden, scientists showed that a little more than a teaspoon of cinnamon added to a bowl of rice pudding lowered the post-meal blood sugar rise in a group of healthy volunteers. These findings were published in the *American Journal of Clinical Nutrition* in 2007.[207]

A study in Pakistan with a small group of people also provides some insight into cinnamon's effect on diabetes. The results demonstrated that subjects who ate one, three, or six grams of cinnamon per day reduced serum glucose (blood sugar), triglyceride, LDL cholesterol, and total cholesterol levels in people with type 2 diabetes. Researchers suggest that including cinnamon in the diet of people with type 2 diabetes will reduce risk factors associated with diabetes and cardiovascular diseases.[208]

Fenugreek

---

[206] Shanmugasundaram KR, Panneerselvam C, Samudram P, Shanmugasundaram ER. Enzyme changes and glucose utilisation in diabetic rabbits: the effect of Gymnema sylvestre, R.Br. J Ethnopharmacol 1983;7:205-234; and Gupta SS, Variyar MC. Experimental studies on pituitary diabetes IV. Effect of Gymnema sylvestre and Coccinia
indica against the hyperglycemia response of somatotropin and corticotrophin hormones. *Indian J Med Res* 1964;52:200-207, and Gupta SS. Inhibitory effect of Gymnema sylvestre (Gurmar) on adrenaline induced hyperglycemia in rats. Indian J Med Sci 1961;15:883-887
[207] Reuters, citing *American Journal of Clinical Nutrition*, June 2007, "Spoonful of Cinnamon Helps the Sugar Go Down," NY, Jun 20, 07
[208] Khan A, Safdar M, Ali Khan MM, Khattak KN, Anderson RA, Cinnamon improves glucose and lipids of people with type 2 diabetes, Department of Human Nutrition, NWFP Agricultural University, Peshawar, Pakistan; *Diabetes Care*, 2003 Dec;26(12):3215-8

Fenugreek, native to the Middle East and India, has been used as a spice and a medicine for thousands of years. Several small pilot studies have suggested that eating five to one hundred grams of fenugreek seeds daily may lower blood glucose levels in both type 1 and type 2 diabetics.[209]

Decades ago, one Indian study reported in the *European Journal of Clinical Nutrition* showed that fenugreek seeds are helpful in the management of diabetes, as they reduced fasting blood sugar and improved glucose tolerance test scores.[210]

Wright State University reports, "Fenugreek seeds have traditionally been used in the treatment of diabetes for centuries. In the last several decades, various well-controlled studies have identified a hypoglycemic [blood sugar-lowering] activity of various fenugreek seed extracts in rabbits, rats, and dogs. While there have been some human studies in India, the size has been too small to come up with a statistically significant result, although they do show that the seed extracts have a hypoglycemic affect in diabetics, which is to say—it lowers the blood sugar."[211]

The Pharmacists Letter Natural Medicines Comprehensive Data Base indicates there are three chemical constituents of fenugreek that affect diabetes. The first is *trigonelline* (also found in coffee) which has a blood sugar–lowering effect as it slows the rate of glucose absorption from the intestinal tract, therefore avoiding spikes in blood levels after meals. Another substance within fenugreek directly appears to stimulate the production of insulin by the pancreas. Fenugreek can be used for both non-insulin-dependent diabetics and insulin-dependent diabetics.[212]

High Chromium Yeast and GTF

Chromium was first identified as a component of the "glucose-tolerance factor" (GTF), required for maintaining normal blood sugar levels. Because the modern diet and commercial farming continues to

---

[209]Schardt, David, Keeping a Lid on Blood Sugar, Nutrition Action Newsletter, May 01, citing Prostaglandins Leukot. Essent. Fatty Acids 56: 379, 1997

[210] Sharma RD, Raghuram TC, Rao NS, Effect of fenugreek seeds on blood glucose and serum lipids in type I diabetes *Eur J Clin Nutr.* 1990 Apr;44(4):301-6; National Institute of Nutrition, Indian Council of Medical Research, Hyderabad.

[211] Wright State University, *Popular Natural Remedies*, Part XVI, Pharmacy Dept., 2003; wright.edu/admin/fredwhite/pharmacy/popular_nremedies16.html

[212] ibid

strip essential nutrients (including minerals) from the soils, our foods just aren't providing us with enough chromium. Nearly thirty years ago, it was discovered that chromium levels in the diet of the United States and Western Europe were lower than our counterparts in the Near and Far East. Tissue levels are also lower in the United States than in other countries.[213] This means we're not gleaning the benefits of much-needed chromium.

Dietary sources of chromium include brewer's yeast, whole grains, potatoes, oysters, liver, seafood, cheese, chicken, and other meat—with brewer's yeast as the richest source of organic chromium complexes.

As part of the GTF molecule, chromium works with insulin to make it possible for cells to move blood sugar out of the blood and into the cells. Chromium may also play a role in other insulin-dependent activities, such as protein and lipid metabolism.[214]

A 1993 study in the Department of Biology at the University of Haifa, Israel, showed conclusive proof that GTF from yeast extract powder decreased blood sugar and free fatty acids in diabetic animals. This, said researchers, proves that GTF has anti-diabetic potential.[215]

Department of Chemistry researchers from the University of Scranton described the benefits of GTF in chromium-rich yeast as instrumental for normal carbohydrate metabolism. When an animal or human is deficient in chromium, the result is an impaired glucose tolerance (problems processing blood sugar).

Scientific experiments have shown that the moment you eat sugar, chromium is moved from where it is stored in your body to work on that sugar. When your diet is filled with refined sugars and carbohydrates, it becomes likely that you're creating a create chromium deficiency, as the mineral is used up in the process of trying to handle the sugar load. Making things worse, because a diet of refined carbohydrates is low in chromium this only and contributes to the

---

[213] Vinson, JA and P Bose, Nutritional Reports International, 30, (4), 1984. THE EFFECT OF A HIGH CHROMIUM YEAST ON THE BLOOD GLUCOSE CONTROL AND BLOOD LIPIDS OF NORMAL AND DIABETIC HUMAN SUBJECTS, Department of Chemistry, University of Scranton, Scranton, PA, 1984
[214] Feinberg School of Medicine, Northwestern University, Chicago, IL, feinberg.northwestern.edu/nutrition/factsheets/chromium.pdf
[215] Mirsky, N, Glucose tolerance factor reduces blood glucose and free fatty acids levels in diabetic rats, J Inorg Biochem, 1993 Feb 1;49(2):123-8, Department of Biology, Oranim, University of Haifa, Tivon, Israel

problem of unstable blood sugar metabolism.[216] In simplest terms, we're not meant to eat so much sugar, and our modern farming methods have destroyed our soils so that they no longer contain enough chromium to address our important health concerns.

---

[216] Vinson, JA, University of Scranton

Cereal Grasses Enrich Your Blood

Green vegetables are great for your health. But why? Certainly, there are great vitamins and minerals. But another part of the secret may be in their chlorophyll, which contains the code for good health; it purifies, cleanses, oxygenates, and enriches the blood. This is one great reason to eat a ton of green foods, including cereal grasses. But don't confuse cereal grasses with breakfast cereals. These are not cereal grasses, but rather processed cereals offering practically no nutritional value.

Barley, alfalfa, wheat grass, and rye—cereal grasses—are often overlooked or ignored as Super Foods, but they are rich in nutrients and chlorophyll.

Food researcher and author Ron Seibold writes:
Many of the components which build and sustain the essential elements in blood are also found in foods that are high in chlorophyll. A remarkable relationship exists between the complex process of respiration in animals and the equally complex but very different process of photosynthesis in plants. In ecological terms, we know that the two processes are interdependent and are essential to the sustenance of all life on Earth. The inhalation of oxygen/expiration of carbon dioxide by animals complements the 'inhalation' of carbon dioxide/expiration of oxygen by plants. The revelation that many of the elements of plant 'blood' resemble and are in some cases identical to those of animal blood is not surprising in this context.

The young cereal plant, dependent on its own rich supply of chlorophyll for the work of growth and development, absorbs and synthesizes the nutrients it requires—vitamin K, vitamin C, folic acid, pyridoxine, iron, calcium and protein. These nutrients are also vital to the generation and utilization of hemoglobin, the energy courier of animal blood. The similarities between chlorophyll and heme are not limited to appearance and function.

Chemists report that the synthesis of heme by animals can occur in much the same way as the synthesis of chlorophyll in plants.[217]

---

[217] Seibold, Ronald, Cereal Grass: What's In It For You?, Pines International, KS, 1990; Shayne, PhD, Vic, Man Cannot Live on Vitamins Alone, 2000

Super Foods & Herbs for Female Health

Mature females are prone to PMS headaches, bloating, breast tenderness, mood swings, and cramps; pre- and post-menopausal symptoms, such as hot flashes, fibroids, osteoporosis, yeast infections, and physical changes that occur from puberty to old age. What's a girl to do? Well, for one thing, plan early on in life for your health. Natural healthcare doctors agree that a diet of organic or biodynamic fruits, seeds, vegetables, nuts, berries, and fish seems to hold the best opportunity for continued health and few symptoms. In today's modern age of artificial ingredients, hormone-laden meats, fluoride, chlorine, and hormone-disrupting and estrogen-mimicking chemicals, a clean diet is a must for ensuring and maintaining superior health.

Following are a few herbs that have been used traditionally for female hormonal problems. Based on the available evidence, evening primrose oil and chasteberry may be reasonable treatment alternatives for some patients with PMS. Dong quai is effective for PMS in many cases, which is why it is used in traditional Chinese multiple-herb formulas.[218]

Chasteberry

Chasteberry, also called *vitex*, is a fruit that grows on a small shrub-like tree native to Central Asia and the Mediterranean region. The name is thought to come from a belief that the plant promoted chastity—because monks in the Middle Ages used chasteberry to decrease sexual desire. However, modern research shows that no clinical data supports using chasteberry for reducing sexual appetite. Chasteberry has traditionally been shown to relieve many female health complaints, especially those relating to menstrual problems.Current scientific literature supports the use of chasteberry for cyclical breast discomfort and premenstrual syndrome.[219]

Beatrix Roemheld-Hamm, MD, PhD, University of Medicine and Dentistry of New Jersey, writes,

---

[218] Hardy, ML, J-Am-Pharm-Assoc-(Wash). 2000 Mar-Apr; 40(2): 234-42; quiz 327-9
[219] Am Fam Physician. 2005 Sep 1;72(5):821-4

Chasteberry has been used for more than 2,500 years to treat various conditions. In ancient Egypt, Greece, and Rome, it was used for a variety of gynecologic conditions. In medieval Europe, chasteberry was popular among celibate clergymen for its purported ability to reduce unwanted sexual libido. Over the past 50 years, chasteberry has been used widely in Europe for gynecologic conditions such as premenstrual syndrome (PMS), cyclical breast discomfort, menstrual cycle irregularities, and dysfunctional uterine bleeding. The German Commission E approves the use of chasteberry for irregularities of the menstrual cycle, cyclical breast discomfort, and PMS, and it is widely prescribed by family physicians and gynecologists in Germany.[220]

Life Extension magazine reports, "Studies have shown that chasteberry acts in the brain to affect the neurotransmitter dopamine, which in turn indirectly affects the release of prolactin. Oscillating prolactin levels are thought to contribute to the breast tenderness and discomfort associated with PMS. Chasteberry has been shown to beneficially regulate several hormones including progesterone."[221]
Chasteberry is thought to have a normalizing effect on the menstrual cycle and has been used successfully to treat both amenorrhea (absence of menstruation) and menorrhagia (heavy menstruation).[222]

Partridge Berry
While the name "squaw vine" is now politically incorrect—and rightly so—this has been the name of a plant used for centuries for women's health issues. Now known as partridge berry or checkerberry, herbalists explain that this herb was used by Native American women to help prepare the body for childbirth and relieve painful menstruation by keeping the uterus toned.[223]

The medicinal uses of partridge berry are not well supported by university research, but the anecdotal evidence for its efficacy is strong.

---

[220] Beatrix Roemheld-Hamm, MD, PhD, University of Medicine and Dentistry of New Jersey, *Journal of the American Academy of Family Physicians*, Sep 1 06
[221] Kiefer, Dale, "A Natural Approach to Menopause," *LE Magazine*, Life Extension Foundation, April 2006
[222] *Integrative Practitioner*, Chasteberry, 2009; integrativepractitioner.net/article_ektid14522.aspx
[223] Grieve, M., Botanical.com, Partridgeberry Profile, hyper-text version of A Modern Herbal, 1931

Many Native American tribes used partridge berry for treating abdominal pain caused by menstrual cramping and for suppressed menstruation. It is now being used by herbalists for the same purposes, as well as for treatment of menstrual pain and for regulating menstrual bleeding.[224]

Dong Quai (also known as Chinese angelica)
Dong quai remains one of the most popular plants in Chinese medicine and is used primarily for gynecological disorders, including painful menstruation or pelvic pain, recovery from childbirth or illness, and fatigue/low vitality. It is also given for strengthening *xue* (loosely translated as "the blood" in Traditional Chinese medicine), for cardiovascular conditions/high blood pressure, inflammation, headache, infections, and nerve pain.[225]

Researchers at the University of Maryland Medical Center report, "Although there are few scientific studies on dong quai, it is sometimes suggested to relieve menstrual disorders such as cramps, irregular menstrual cycles, infrequent periods, premenstrual syndrome, and menopausal symptoms."[226]

When taking dong quai, a number of women have reported relief from symptoms such as hot flashes. Researchers aren't sure whether dong quai has estrogen-like effects or if it blocks estrogens in the body, and the studies so far have been conflicting.[227] One explanation may be that it, like most other Chinese herbs, is used as a means of balancing the system, rather than having the effects of stimulating or suppressing symptoms that are associated with modern drug therapy.

Since much of the discomfort with female health problems involving PMS and menstruation is associated with inflammation, researchers at the Department of Pharmacology at the University of Hong Kong studied the effects of polysaccharides isolated in dong quai

---

[224] The Herbal Dispatch, Vol6 No6, Mountain State University, Beckley, WV, Aug 2008

[225] US National Library of Medicine, National Institutes of Health, Bethesda, MD Aug 09

[226] University of Maryland Medical Center, umm.edu/altmed/articles/dong-quai-000238.htm

[227] ibid

as they relate to gastrointestinal damage. It became clear that the herb possesses protective anti-inflammatory properties.[228]

Black Cohosh

Life Extension magazine reports that black cohosh is effective in reducing the severity, duration, and incidence of hot flashes and night sweats."[229]

Black cohosh has also been cited as improving menopause-associated symptoms of anxiety and depression. In one study, effects were noted within the first month of treatment and continued in its usefulness for the three-month duration of the study.[230]

One of the major concerns associated with aging women is the threat of osteoporosis, or bone loss, due to declining estrogen levels. Unfortunately, modern medical attempts to ameliorate osteoporosis by using hormone replacement therapy. The downside to this approach is an increased risk of cancer.

In laboratory experiments, black cohosh prevented bone loss following removal of the ovaries of lab animals. Black cohosh did not appear to adversely affect the uterus, which may account for its superior safety profile compared to hormone replacement therapy. Black cohosh not only reduces hot flashes, anxiety, and depression in menopausal women, but also appears to prevent some of the bone loss associated with the natural decline in estrogens, without the risk of stimulating uterine or breast cancer that is presented by drugs.[231]

---

[228] Cho CH, Mei QB, Shang P, Lee SS, So HL, Guo X, Li Y. Study of the gastrointestinal protective effects of polysaccharides from Angelica sinensis in rats. *Planta Med.* 2000 May; 66(4): 348-51, cited in Nutraceutical Library, nutraceuticallibrary.com, 09

[229] Kiefer, Dale, "A Natural Approach to Menopause," *LE Magazine*, Life Extension Foundation, April 2006

[230] ibid, citing Pockaj BA, Loprinzi CL, Sloan JA, et al. Pilot evaluation of black cohosh for the treatment of hot flashes in women. *Cancer Invest.* 2004;22(4):515-21, and Nappi RE, Malavasi B, Brundu B, Facchinetti F. Efficacy of Cimicifuga racemosa on climacteric complaints: a randomized study versus low-dose transdermal estradiol. *Gynecol Endocrinol.* 2005 Jan;20(1):30-5

[231] ibid, citing Seidlova-Wuttke D, Hesse O, Jarry H, et al. Evidence for selective estrogen receptor modulator activity in a black cohosh (Cimicifuga racemosa) extract: comparison with estradiol-17beta. Eur J Endocrinol. 2003 Oct;149(4):351-62

More Foods For Female Health

Looking into our research files, we've found a number of interesting correlations between some female hormonal symptoms and missing nutrients.

Certainly, it's better to improve your diet and lifestyle *before* you get the headaches, cramps, dizziness, food cravings, insomnia, crying spells, nausea, or irritability. Some of the worst offenders include bad fats (omega-3 fats are good choices), sugar, non-organic meats (hormones in meat can affect your hormonal system), lack of daily exercise that's vigorous enough to increase your heart rate and burn calories, as well as avoidance of toxic substances in personal care products, bug sprays, plastics, and so forth. As we have discussed already in this book, there are several herbs and foods that benefit the female hormonal system. But this chapter takes a look at some possible mineral and vitamin deficiencies that links to female problems.

Stephen Byrnes, ND, author of *The Lazy Person's Guide to Whole Foods Cooking,* writes, "Natural therapists have long thought that the root of premenstrual syndrome is biochemical, resulting ultimately in hormonal imbalance. Today it is axiomatic that PMS is a condition of excess estrogen with a corresponding deficiency of progesterone."[232]

Fish Oils

There are two main types of cramping associated with the menstrual cycle: spasmodic and congestive. Essential fatty acids of the omega-3 variety are helpful with cramps and pain. In fact, women may often be able to take less of their prescription drugs when supplementing their diet with fish oil.[233]

---

[232] Byrnes, ND, Stephen, Natural PMS Relief, Weston A. Price quarterly newsletter, winter 2000

[233] Complementary, supplementary and non-medical interventions for menstrual pain, University of Maryland School of Medicine, Integrative Medicine, Menstrual Pain, Cochrane Reviews, medschool.umaryland.edu/integrative/cochrane-reviews/cochrane-rev-menstrual.asp , 09

Uterine cramping is one of the most common uncomfortable sensations women can experience during menstruation. A speculated cause for spasmodic cramping is prostaglandins, which are chemicals responsible for the relaxation and contraction of muscles. A diet high in essential fatty acids (found in vegetables and fish) increases the prostaglandins for aiding muscle relaxation. Congestive cramping causes the body to retain fluids and salt. To counter it, avoid wheat products, dairy products, alcohol, caffeine, and refined sugar.[234]

Magnesium And Headaches

It has been estimated that 70 percent of migraine sufferers are female. Of these, 60 to 70 percent report that their migraines come with their menstrual cycles. "Premenstrual migraines regularly occur during or after the time when the female hormones, estrogen and progesterone, decrease to their lowest levels."[235]

Magnesium may help relieve headaches,[236] especially because it has a relaxing effect on muscles and blood vessels. Studies show that about half of migraine headache sufferers have a low amount of ionized magnesium in the blood, which suggests a low magnesium status. And magnesium supplementation reduces the number and duration of migraines, including menstrual migraines, in some people. The findings suggest that too little magnesium can worsen the suffering from migraine headaches.[237]

Calcium And Vitamin D

Studies suggest that calcium levels are lower in women experiencing PMS, and that calcium supplements may reduce the severity of such symptoms, including anxiety, loneliness, irritability, tearfulness, and tension. One study conducted by Dr. Elizabeth R. Bertone-Johnson and her colleagues at the University of Massachusetts–Amherst involved

---

[234] Menstrual Cycles:
What Really Happens in those 28 Days?! Feminist Womens Health Center, Seattle, WA, fwhc.org, May 09
[235] Migraines, Headaches, and Hormones, webmd.com/migraines-headaches/guide/hormones-headaches
[236] Facchinetti F, Sances G, Borella P, Genazzani AR, Nappi G., Magnesium prophylaxis of menstrual migraine: effects on intracellular magnesium, University Centre for Adaptive Disorders and Headache (UCADH), Dept. of Obstetrics and Gynecology, Italy; Headache. 1991 May;31(5):298-301
[237] Nielsen, Forrest H, Migraines, Sleeplessness, Heart Attacks — Magnesium? USDA Agricultural Research Service, Oct 06

over a thousand women with PMS and close to two thousand women without PMS. The results showed that women with the highest vitamin D intake—amounting to approximately 400iu per day from food sources—were less likely to experience PMS compared to those with the lowest intake. Adequate amounts of calcium in the diet, approximating about 1200mg a day, were also shown to be effective in relieving PMS.[238] The secret here seems to be getting enough of both calcium and vitamin D together, because they have a synergistic effect in the body.

Calcium has the capacity to improve mood swings, pain, bloating, depression, back pain, and food cravings, so it's worth considering your intake if you have PMS problems.[239]

Vitamin B Complex

Because vitamin B foods offer so many benefits to the body—from nerve transmission to energy production — the vitamin B complex is helpful when dealing with most menstrual problems, which are complex in their origins.

One good source of the vitamin B complex is brewer's yeast, which, by the way, has no relationship to yeast infections, despite what uninformed sources on the Internet may report. Brewer's yeast should be taken in moderate amounts because some people have reported headaches after taking large doses of it. However, you shouldn't get a headache if you're taking brewer's yeast in a whole food supplement and eating a healthy diet full of other nutritional foods.

Brewer's yeast is a rich source of minerals, including chromium—an essential trace mineral that helps the body maintain normal blood sugar levels, selenium, and protein. B-complex vitamins in brewer's yeast include B1 (thiamine), B2 (riboflavin), B3 (niacin), B5 (pantothenic acid), B6 (pyridoxine), B9 (folic acid), and H or B7 (biotin). These vitamins help break down carbohydrates, fats, and proteins, to provide the body with energy. The vitamin B complex also feeds the nervous system, helps maintain muscles used for digestion, and keeps skin, hair, eyes, mouth, and liver healthy. Vitamin B12, an essential vitamin found in meat and dairy products is not found in

---

[238] Arch Intern Med. 2005; 165:1246-1252

[239] Thys-Jacobs S, Starkey P, Bernstein D, et al. Calcium carbonate and the premenstrual syndrome: effects on premenstrual and menstrual symptoms. Premenstrual Syndrome Study Group. Am J Obstet Gynecol. 1998;179:444-452.

brewer's yeast; vegetarians sometimes take brewer's yeast mistakenly, believing that it provides this important part of the vitamin complex.[240]

---

[240] University of Maryland Medical Center, umm.edu/altmed/articles/brewers-yeast-000288.htm, 09

Super Foods For Him

It's no secret that men are more likely to neglect their health than women are. The American Academy of Family Physicians (AAFP) reports that nearly 30 percent of men say they wait "as long as possible" before seeking help when they feel sick, are in pain, or are concerned about their health.[241] We can only suspect that this number has risen in recent years due to the numbers of people who cannot afford health insurance.

Men in the United States may not be as healthy as they say they are. The survey showed that they spend an average of nineteen hours a week watching television and more than four hours a week watching sports, but just slightly more than a third (38 percent) of men exercise on a regular basis. And, the Centers for Disease Control (CDC) in Washington, D.C. estimates that nearly three-quarters (71 percent) of men are overweight. "One of the biggest obstacles to improving the health of men is men themselves," said Rick Kellerman, MD, president of the AAFP. "They don't make their health a priority. Fortunately, 78 percent of the men with a spouse or significant other surveyed say their spouse or significant other has some influence over their decision to go to the doctor."[242]

What can men do to be healthier? The same thing as women when it comes to their daily diet—more real foods and no junk foods, artificial ingredients, bad fats, or sugars. Of course, there are specific health concerns that women do not encounter that cause men a lot of concern, including (but not limited to) erectile dysfunction, testicular and prostate cancer, loss of sexual desire, sterility, and more.

Experts say that if you're a man and you live long enough, you'll most likely develop benign prostatic hyperplasia (BPH), which is a medical term for an enlarged prostate. Ninety percent of men show signs of such prostatic enlargement by age eighty. Symptoms may

---

[241] Lee, Adam, New Survey Finds Majority of Men Avoid Preventive Health Measures, American Academy of Family Physicians, news release, June 19, 2007
[242] ibid

include dribbling after urination, referred pain to the penis, and the impulse to get up many times during the night to urinate.

Men should know about a few foods that have been shown to address specific male-oriented health concerns...

Guava Seed

Guava was domesticated in Peru several thousands of years ago. Peruvian archaeological sites turned up guava seeds that were stored with beans, corn, squash, and other cultivated plants, so they know guava was a part of the ancient diet. Laboratory study shows that guava is rich in tannins, phenols, triterpenes, flavonoids, essential oils, saponins, carotenoids, lectins, vitamins, fiber, and fatty acids.

Medical research shows guava seed to be one of the best sources of lycopene, an antioxidant shown to offer protection against prostate cancer. Lycopene, one of over six hundred carotenoids, is one of the main carotenoids found in human plasma. As mentioned earlier, lycopene is responsible for the red coloring of various foods (guava, red grapefruit, watermelon, etc.). Lycopene is a natural pigment produced by plants and microorganisms (but not animals) and is one of the most potent antioxidants—twice as effective as that of beta-carotene and ten times higher than that of alpha-tocopherol.[243]

Studies based either on dietary supplement intake or blood/tissue measurements of carotenoids have been the primary methods used to identify lycopene's role in lowering the risk of developing or enhancing the growth of prostate cancer cells.

Saw Palmetto

Saw palmetto is a type of palm tree that grows in the southeastern United States. It is native to the Southern Atlantic coast through the Gulf coast, from South Carolina through Texas. The berry from this tree has long been used in Native American healing and enjoyed a role in treatment of prostate and other urinary problems from the 1870s until around 1950. After that point, saw palmetto lost its drug status and came to be seen as merely an herb. However, saw palmetto is still used in Europe as a treatment for benign prostate hypertrophy (BPH)—non-cancerous swelling of the prostate gland. It's been approved by the

---

[243] Sanjiv A and Rao, AV. Tomato lycopene and its role in human health and chronic diseases. Canadian Medical Association Journal, Volume 163(6):739-744, September 19, 2000

German Commission E, an official body that evaluates herbal treatments for their safety and to assess well they work.[244]   Saw palmetto berries contain lauric and other fatty acids, phytosterols, polysaccharides, and monoacylglycerides, which are anti-inflammatory and prostatic (prostate) cell proliferation chemicals.[245] Saw palmetto contains a combination of anti-androgenic (hormone-balancing) and anti-inflammatory actions. It helps to increase urinary flow in men with enlarged prostates, but it does not decrease the size of the prostate gland.[246]

Some medical research shows that saw palmetto's effects are like those of a prescription drug used for BPH, called Finasteride (commonly used for hair loss). While both Finasteride and saw palmetto may improve a man's ability to urinate by allowing urine to flow out of the bladder faster and reducing the number of times he needs to get up during the night to urinate, saw palmetto is safer and without the drug's side effects.

Pumpkin Seed

The *Indian Journal of Urology* states, "Besides having a pleasant flavor, pumpkin seeds are known to possess antidepressant properties in Chinese history. More importantly, pumpkin seed ingestion can influence positively prostate health, which is very important for male sexual health. It is commonly used to strengthen the prostate gland and promote healthy hormone function in men. Myosin, an amino acid found in pumpkin seeds, is known to be essential for muscular contractions."[247]

---

[244] Saw Palmetto - Topic Overview; men.webmd.com/tc/saw-palmetto-topic-overview, 2009

[245] Long, Scott F, RPh, PhD, Assistant Professor of Pharmacology & Toxicology, *Herbal Supplements*
An Overview of the Pharmacognosy, Pharmacology, Clinical Therapeutics and Use of Selected Herbal Products, Southwestern Oklahoma State University Weatherford, OK, 2009

[246] *Popular Natural Remedies*, Wright State University, Dept of Pharmacy, Daton, OH, 2009

[247] Peter Lim Huat Chy, Department of Urology, Changi General Hospital, Singapore; Adjunct Professor, Edith Cowan University, Australia, Traditional Asian folklore medicines in sexual health, *The Indian Journal of Urology*, 2006, citing Rowland DL, Tai W. A review of plant-derived and herbal approaches to the treatment of sexual dysfunctions. *J Sex Marital Ther* 2003;29:185-205

Utah State University researchers report, "Pumpkin and pumpkin seeds are high in vitamin A, protein, fiber, zinc, iron and monounsaturated and polyunsaturated fat. Health benefits of eating pumpkin include: healthy cardiovascular system (mono and polyunsaturated fats), healthy skin (vitamin A), healthy vision (vitamin A), decreased osteoporosis (zinc), decreased arthritis (less lipid peroxidation), decreased prostate enlargement (helps prevent conversion of testosterone to dihydrotestosterone) and decreased colon cancer (fiber)."[248]

It appears that the medical jury is still out when it comes to deciding whether pumpkin seeds have a beneficial effect on prostate disease and symptoms. However, when combined with saw palmetto in a Swedish study, results were promising. The study showed better urinary flow and improved frequency of urination.[249]

Licorice Root
Licorice root is part of a purple and white, flowering perennial plant that's related to the pea, originally from the Mediterranean region and central and southwest Asia. Traditionally, it's been boiled to extract its sweetness, which has been popularized in licorice candy. But licorice root also serves as a powerful and effective herbal medicine. Licorice was used in ancient Greece, China, and Egypt—mainly for gastritis (inflammation of the stomach) and ailments of the upper respiratory tract. Ancient Egyptians made a licorice drink for ritual use to honor spirits of the pharaohs. And medicinally, licorice use became widespread in Europe and Asia for numerous indications.[250]

As of late, researchers discovered that licorice exhibits a powerful influence over cancer cells in the prostate gland.[251] Kimberly M. Jackson, assistant professor of chemistry at Spelman College in Atlanta, first discovered the ability of licorice root compound to inhibit prostate cancer.[252] Research shows that licorice root causes the death of

---

[248] Hinkamp, Dennis, Ask a specialist: What are the health benefits of pumpkin? Nothing Scary About Pumpkins' Nutrition, Utah State University, Extension News & Multimedia; Oct 9, 2008
[249] Br J Urol. 1990 Dec;66(6):639-41
[250] Licorice (Glycyrrhiza glabra L.) and DGL (deglycyrrhizinated licorice), National Library of Medicine, Bethesda, MD, 2009
[251] J. Agric. Food Chem., 2009, 57 (18), pp 8266–8273
[252] Darcey, Julia, A Natural Product Gives Hope for Slowing Prostate Cancer, MBL Visiting Researcher Kimberly Jackson studies how a compound from licorice root works in prostate cancer cells, Marine Biology Laboratory, August 17, 2009

prostate cancer cells, and it continues to be studied for other benefits, including how it protects the liver and works against tumors.

Ginseng Root

If you're concerned about prostate cancer, ginseng is an herb you'll want to know about. Ginseng is another plant that has been used since ancient times—as an aphrodisiac, a tonic for well-being, and as a curative medicine for a variety of illnesses. In animal studies, ginseng was used to regulate hormone levels and positively affect the prostate gland.[253] Other studies show that ginseng inhibits prostate cancer.[254]

Ginseng root and its active ingredients have been associated with a wide range of biological activities, such as anti-diabetic immune stimulation and an ability to stop or slow down the growth of a variety of cultured cancer cells. The exact way that ginseng and ginsenosides work to kill cancer cells is not entirely clear, but their interaction with the cell membranes leading to the destruction of the strength of cancer cell walls is well known to researchers.[255]

Pygeum

The pygeum tree is a tall evergreen that grows in central and southern Africa. Its bark has been used since ancient times to treat problems relating to urination.

Biologist Kristine Stewart, Department of Biological Sciences, Florida International University, wrote, "I studied the uses of the African cherry (*Prunus africana*) by four ethnic groups who live near the Kilum-Ijim Forest Preserve on Mount Oku, Cameroon...[I]ts greatest value is for traditional medicines. Healers use the bark and leaves to treat more than thirty human ailments and several animal diseases and it is the most important plant used in their practices." With her study, Stewart set out to be the first to document the importance of pygeum, particularly for animal medicines. She wrote, "I also

---

[253] *Arch Androl.* 1982 Jun;8(4):261-3

[254] Liu WK, Xu SX, Che CT, Department of Anatomy, Faculty of Medicine, The Chinese University of Hong Kong, Shatin, New Territories, Anti-proliferative effect of ginseng saponins on human prostate cancer cell line., *Life Sci.* 2000 Aug 4;67(11):1297-306

[255] Popovich, David G., Shi Yun Yeo and Wei Zhang, Ginseng (Panax quinquefolius) and Licorice (Glycyrrhiza uralensis) Root Extract Combinations Increase Hepatocarcinoma Cell (Hep-G2) Viability, Department of Chemistry, National University of Singapore, Singapore, Oxford Journals, Evidence-based Complementary and Alternative Medicine, 2009

examined the growing worldwide herbal use to treat benign prostatic hyperplasia. At least seventeen double blind trials of pygeum for BPH have been performed, involving a total of almost a thousand individuals and ranging in length from forty-five to ninety days. Many of these studies were poorly reported and/or designed. Nonetheless, overall the results make a meaningful case that pygeum can reduce symptoms such as nighttime urination, urinary frequency, and residual urine volume."[256]

Studies were conducted in several places throughout Europe and included nearly three-hundred men between the ages of fifty and eighty-five. Participants received 50 mg of a pygeum extract or placebo twice daily. The results showed significant improvements in residual urine volume, voided volume, urinary flow rate, nighttime urination, and daytime frequency. But scientists still say they do not know how pygeum works. Yet, unlike the drug Finasteride, pygeum is thought to reduce inflammation in the prostate, and to inhibit prostate growth factors, substances implicated in problematic prostate enlargement.[257]

---

[256] Stewart, Kristine M, The African Cherry (Prunus africana): from Hoe-Handles to the International herb market, Department of Biological Sciences, Florida International University, University Park, Miami, FL, Economic Botany 57(4):559-569. 2003; doi: 10.1663/0013-0001(2003)057[0559:TACPAF]2.0.CO;2

[257] ibid

Immune-Bolstering Super Foods

Entire books have been written about the immune system, so we won't even attempt to delve into the details of this very complex subject. Instead, let's take a look at some highlights.

The immune system is just this—a system. This means that no singular organ, gland, or cell holds the key to keeping your body safe from illness or injury. Protecting your body is a cooperative enterprise between the good bacteria in your digestive tract, killer T-cells in your blood stream, white blood cells, lymph nodes, oxygen, protective skin cells, enzymes, and a lot more. The immune system is a "team approach" within the body, involved with preventing illness, fighting off foreign invaders (including toxins), and protecting native cells.

If you imagine your body as a fortified castle, then you can appreciate the importance of defending against foreign invaders always threatening to attack and interfere with the functions going on within the castle walls. Biologically, the castle is you and your immune system. And the attackers come in the forms of viruses, bacteria, damaged DNA, stagnancy, free-radical molecules, injuries, pollution, poisons, and more. There are so many attackers that it takes a full-time "army" to wage a successful defense. Failure to do so can result in any number of problems, ranging from the common cold to cancer, from out-of-control infections to AIDS, and from chronic fatigue to gum disease. The stronger your immune system is, the better it fights for your good health.

Various foods and herbs are especially heralded in supporting the immune system. Good sources include acerola berries, astragalus, carrots, garlic, Maitake mushrooms, green tea leaves, echinacea, and American or Asian ginseng root. In fact, most fruits and vegetables are highly protective and detoxifying because they contain phytochemicals that stimulate the immune system, eliminate toxins, and even destroy microbes.

Acerola Berry

Native to the Amazon rainforest, acerola berries are ten to fifty times higher in vitamin C than oranges, pound for pound. The fruit is valued for its anti-free radicals and antioxidant properties.

Astragalus

As one of the most powerful immune-system supporters, the Super Food astragalus is mentioned a few places in this book. Herbalist Rob MacCaleb writes, "Astragalus stimulates virtually every phase of immune system activity. It increases the number of 'stem cells' in the marrow and lymph tissue and stimulates their development into active immune cells, which are released into the body. Research documenting this also demonstrated that astragalus could promote or trigger immune cells from the 'resting' state into heightened activity."[258]

Maitake Mushroom

Maitake mushroom is another powerful immune-boosting food. The active constituent is thought to be a beta-glucan polysaccharide, which, among other benefits, helps fight cancer and keeps it from spreading throughout the body.[259] According to researchers at Memorial Sloan-Kettering Cancer Center, the Maitake mushroom is believed to possess the ability to activate various effector cells (important cells that perform when they are stimulated to do so), such as macrophages, natural killer cells, and T cells.[260]

Researchers from the University of Alabama A&M Department of Agriculture report:

> Maitake is a fungus that grows most frequently on fallen trees or stumps of beech and oak….In traditional Chinese medicine, it has been used for improving spleen and stomach ailments, calming nerves, and treating hemorrhoids (Hobbs, 1995; Jong and Birmingham, 1990). Recent studies have shown that polysaccharides and polysaccharide-protein complexes from this mushroom have significant anti-cancer activity (Hishida et al., 1988; Kurashige et al., 1997; Ohno et al., 1985). Other fractions (D-, GF-1, grifolan-7N) from maitake exhibit immunological enhancement together with properties of anti-

---

[258] MacCaleb, Rob, "Boosting Immunity With Herbs," .ibiblio.org/herbs/immune; Herb Research Foundation; citing Mavligit, G.M. et al., 1979, J. Immunology, 123, pp. 2185-88 and Chu, D., et al., Clin. Immuno. and Immunopathology, 1987, 45, pp. 48-57. Chu, D., et al., J. Clin. Lab. Immunol., 1988, 25, 125-9.

[259] Kodama N, Komuta K, Nanba H. Can Maitake MD-fraction aid cancer patients? Altern Med Rev 2002;7:236-9.

[260] mskcc.org/mskcc/html/69294.cfm#References

HIV, antihypertension, antidiabetic, and antiobesity (Adachi et al., 1988; Borchers et al., 1999; Iino et al., 1985; Jones, 1998; Kabir et al., 1987; Kubo et al, 1994; Kubo and Nanba, 1966; Mizuno and Zhuang, 1995; Nakai et al., 1999; Nanba, 1993). The ß-glucan fractions from this mushroom are now being used by over 3,000 health professionals in the United States for the prevention and treatment of flu and common infection, AIDS (HIV), diabetes mellitus, hypertension, hypercholesterolemia, and urinary tract infections (Choi et al., 2001; Cichoke, 1994; Kabir et al., 1989; Kubo et al.,1997; Kubo et al., 1994; Smith, 2002; Talpur, 2002).

...Several studies have been conducted to measure maitake's effect on obesity. In animal studies, lack of weight gain or weight loss was significant (Ohtsuru, 1992). In an obesity study on humans by Dr. Yokota (1992), 30 patients were given a powdered maitake food supplement for two months with no change in their regular diets. All patients successfully lost 7-13 pounds.

Maitake, as is true of many other mushrooms, is predominately an immune booster. The human body uses these high-molecular-weight polysaccharides to enhance its immune system. [M]uch of the research suggests that Maitake and other mushrooms, taken along with traditional therapy, provides improved response and recovery as well as protecting healthy cells from cancer.[261]

In a study led by Dr. Hiroaki Nanba of Kobe Pharmaceutical University in Japan,[262] researchers demonstrated that Maitake powder and MD Fraction, its advanced extract, enhances immune cell activity and helps fight cancer. They reported that "cancer regression or significant symptom improvement was observed in 58.3 percent of liver cancer patients, 68.8 percent of breast cancer patients, and 62.5 percent of lung cancer patients. Furthermore, when Maitake was taken

---

[261] Sabota, Cathy, Maitake Mushrooms for Your Health, Metro News, Alabama Cooperative Extension Program, Universities of Alabama A&M and Auburn, aces.edu/urban/metronews/vol4no1/mushroom.html, 2009
[262] Altern Med Rev 2002;7(3):236-239

in addition to chemotherapy, immune-competent cell activities were enhanced 1.2-1.4 times, compared with chemotherapy alone."[263]

Green Tea

Green tea comes from the leaves of a plant that has been consumed since ancient times as not only a pleasant-tasting beverage, but also as a medicinal herb in the Orient and Asia. Topically, it has been used effectively to treat genital and perianal warts, among other skin problems.[264] The anticancer effect of green tea has been credited to its ample supply of polyphenols (types of antioxidants found in many natural plant foods).[265]

Echinacea

Echinacea is a plant that grows wild in various parts of the world. You may even mistake it for a purple-flowered weed. Its stigma, consisting of a bright, round bulb, earned the plant its befitting nickname, "coneflower." Echinacea was shown by researchers to stimulate phagocytosis (the cellular "eating" of debris and foreign invaders within the body), enhance mobility of leukocytes (cells of the immune system defending the body against both infectious disease and foreign materials), stimulate TNF (tumor necrosis factor, keeping cells in check) and interleukin 1 (special immune cells) secretion from other immune cells (including those in the lymphatic system), and improve respiratory activity.[266] If that's too much science for you, just remember echinacea is a plant that has been used by everyone from Native American herbalists to modern nutritionists for a medley of ailments, including tumors, snakebites, infections, and the common cold.

Herbalist-author James Duke, PhD, reports that there's been a good amount of research to show that echinacea strengthens the immune system against cold viruses and many other germs. He notes that echinacea "increases levels of a chemical in the body called

---

[263] Maitake given go-ahead for human drug trials, Nutra-ingredients-usa, Decision News Media SAS, Ap 1 04

[264] Memorial Sloan Kettering Cancer Center website, citing Stockfleth E, et al. Topical Polyphenon E in the treatment of external genital and perianal warts: a randomized controlled trial. *Br J Dermatol.* Jun 2008;158(6):1329-1338.

[265] Tosetti F, Ferrari N, De Flora S. Angioprevention: angiogenesis is a common and key target for cancer chemopreventive agents. FASEB J 2002;16:2-14; and Yang CS, et al. Prevention of carcinogenesis by tea polyphenols. *Drug Metab Rev* 2001;33:237-53.

[266] Memorial Sloan Kettering Cancer Center, "Echinacea," mskcc.org/mskcc/html/69209.cfm, 2009

properdin, which activates the part of the immune system responsible for increasing defense mechanisms against viruses and bacteria. Echinacea root extracts also possess antiviral activity against influenza, herpes and other viruses."[267]

Ginseng

American and Asian ginseng varieties belong to the genus Panax and have similar chemical compositions. Siberian ginseng (also known as Eleuthero) belongs to *Eleutherococcus,* a different genus from American and Asian ginsengs, thus rendering it an entirely different plant that does not contain ginsenosides, the active ingredients found in Asian and American ginsengs. However, all three ginsengs are adaptogens—substances that strengthen the body, helping it return to normal when it's been subjected to prolonged stress. This makes ginseng beneficial for those recovering from illness or surgery, especially the elderly who tend to have less energy and capacity for recovery than younger people.[268]

American and Asian ginsengs show promise for treating cancer, regulating blood sugar metabolism, addressing Alzheimer's Disease, helping with attention deficit disorder, and bolstering weak immune systems. University of Maryland Medical Center pharmacists report, "Studies suggest that regular intake of ginseng may reduce one's chances of getting various types of cancer, especially lung, liver, stomach, pancreatic and ovarian. A laboratory study found that American ginseng may also enhance the effects of medications used to treat breast cancer, potentially allowing the doctor to use less chemotherapy."[269]

Adding to this, James Duke, PhD, writes, "Commission E, the group of scientists that advises the German government about herbs, endorses ginseng 'as a tonic to combat feelings of lassitude and debility, lack of energy and ability to concentrate, and during convalescence'...Clinical studies indicate that ginseng improves athletic performance...and stimulates the immune system, an effect that's been repeatedly confirmed in experiments with animals."[270]

---

[267] Duke, PhD, James, The Green Pharmacy, p. 135
[268] Ernest B. Hawkins, MS, BSPharm, RPh, Health Education Resources; and Steven D. Ehrlich, NMD, "American Ginseng," University of Maryland Medical Center, 2007
[269] ibid
[270] Duke, PhD, James, The Green Pharmacy, p. 132

Top Immune Boosters

There are actions you can take to boost your immune system, but here are the top five, incorporating not only Super Foods, but lifestyle and dietary changes as well:

1. Support the gut. It's said that your immune system begins in your digestive tract. This is true. There are bacteria in your intestines that break down food and protect your body from illness. When you take antibiotics or eat an excessive amount of sugar and processed foods, the good bacteria in your intestines cannot do their job to protect and defend your body. You may want to begin taking some probiotics (good bacteria) in the form of acidophilus if you have digestive difficulties, yeast infections, jock itch, fungus, or a sluggish immune system. You'll find probiotics in the refrigerated section of your local health food store.

2. Keep your body out of extreme temperatures. If your mother ever told you to dress warm, maybe she was paying attention to what doctors have been saying about the cold shocking our bodies. When we're exposed to extreme temperatures, our immune systems are challenged. As the weather continues to slide into the wintry months, dress warm and protect your head, chest, and neck. And when it gets hot, let your body adjust to a cooler temperature before stepping into a cold building or turning the air conditioning in your car to full blast.

3. Sleep well. Sleep is the great restorer of energy. All creatures do it, and you're a creature, so you should do it, too. Turn off your television, read, then fall asleep. Your immune system will love you for it!

4. Eat immune-supporting foods and herbs. Some of the best include (in no particular order) Maitake mushroom, broccoli, garlic, acerola berry, garlic, astralagus, carrots, green tea, echinacea, Siberian ginseng, wheat germ, apples, kelp, and a wide variety of fruits, berries, nuts, seeds, and vegetables. George L. Blackburn, MD, PhD, associate director of the nutrition division at Harvard Medical School in Boston, said, "Nutrition plays an important part in maintaining immune function. Insufficiency in one or more essential nutrients may prevent the immune system from functioning at its peak."[271]

5. Exercise Regularly. Moving your limbs and body around stimulates your lymphatic system, increases your heart rate, boosts your circulation, expands your lung capacity, and relieves stress.

There are more actions you can take and certain foods you may eat, but if you begin with these top five, you'll be on your way to protecting the system that protects the rest of you!

---

[271] "Follow this eat-right plan to fortify your immune system," cnn.com, 2008

Feeding Your Liver

The liver is the largest organ inside the body, and it plays a vital role in performing many complex functions that are essential for life. Your liver serves as your body's internal chemical-manufacturing plant. While there are still many things we do not understand about the workings of the liver, we do know that it's impossible to live without it and that its well-being is a major factor in the quality of your life. By adding certain Super Foods to your diet, you can not only support the health of your liver, but also all of its functions.

Signs Of Liver Problems

Many people are not aware of common symptoms of liver problems. Chronic fatigue and feeling tired after meals, as well as depression, mood instability, and irrational anger and temper flare-ups may be liver related. Even PMS symptoms, including breast soreness and sensitivity, low blood sugar, and irritability may be due to liver problems. In the early 1940s, Morton Biskind, MD, published several articles in endocrinology journals linking PMS to a B-vitamin and protein deficiencies in the diet. These deficiencies led to the liver's difficulty in de-activating estrogen.

Other liver-related symptoms may include nausea, a problem digesting and utilizing fats, foul-smelling gas, swollen belly, loss of appetite, constipation, and diarrhea. Aching joints and muscles, sore feet, psoriasis, and slow wound healing are other signs of a problematic liver. Headaches (especially behind the eyes), insomnia, difficulty awakening, poor memory, and difficulty concentrating are possible symptoms showing a dysfunction between the brain and the liver.[272]

Some Important Liver Functions Include:
- Converting food into stored energy and chemicals that are necessary for life and growth
- Filtering alcohol, drugs, and other toxic substances out of the blood and converting them into substances that can be excreted from the body

---

[272] http://www.hepatitis.org.uk/s-crina/liver-f3-main3.htm

- Manufacturing and exporting important body chemicals, such as hormones, vitamin A, vitamin B12, digestive enzymes, etc.
- Converting food nutrients for utilization—85 to 90 percent of the blood that leaves the stomach and intestines carries important nutrients to the liver
- Processing carbohydrates, proteins, fats, and minerals so that they can be used to maintain normal body functions

Carbohydrates, or sugars, are stored as glycogen in the liver and are released as energy between meals, or when the body's energy demands are high. In this way, the liver helps to regulate your blood sugar level and prevent chronic hypoglycemia (low blood sugar). This enables us to keep an even level of energy throughout the day. Without this balance, we would need to eat constantly to keep up our energy.

Once in the liver, proteins are released to the muscles as energy, stored for later use, or converted to urea for excretion in the urine. Certain proteins are converted into ammonia (a toxic metabolic product) by bacteria in the intestine or during the breakdown of body protein. The ammonia must be broken down by the liver and made into urea, which is then excreted by the kidneys. The liver also has the unique ability to convert certain amino acids into sugar for quick energy.

Fats cannot be digested without bile, which is made in the liver, stored in the gallbladder, and released (as needed) into the small intestine. Bile acids act like a detergent, breaking apart fats and oils into much smaller droplets so they can be acted upon by intestinal enzymes and absorbed. Bile is also essential for the absorption of vitamins A, D, E, and K, the fat-soluble vitamins. After digestion, bile acids are reabsorbed by the intestine, returned to the liver, and recycled as bile once again.

What Is "Fatty Liver" And Is It Caused By Eating Too Much Fat?
"Fatty liver" is not a disease, but rather a pathological finding. A more appropriate term would be "fatty infiltration of the liver," a condition which isn't caused by eating too many fats. Nutritional causes of fatty infiltration of the liver include starvation, obesity, protein malnutrition, and intestinal bypass operation for obesity. Fatty liver can also be caused by endocrine disorders, or a buildup of certain chemical or drug compounds in the body. Such drugs can be prescription, over-the-counter, or recreational.

Coffee Enema For Liver Detoxification

Coffee enemas have been used by a number of natural healthcare practitioners, including Dr. Gerson at his cancer treatment center, as a means of detoxifying the liver. Used in this way, caffeine causes your gallbladder to empty the toxins in its liver ducts and move them out through the bowels for elimination. The alkaloids in the caffeine stimulate the production of an enzyme called "glutathione-S-transferase," an enzyme that facilitates the liver detoxification pathways.

Foods That Hurt

Common foods can lead to liver problems, including excess coffee, any food that contains pesticide residues (non-organic foods), junk foods, and artificial fats (such as margarine, trans-fats, refined sugars, french fries, fried chicken, doughnuts, and chips). Frequent consumption of alcohol can lead to a fatty liver as well.

Super Foods That Heal

Dark green, leafy vegetables support liver health, as well as parsley, turmeric, radishes, licorice (not the candy), kale, garlic, beets, carrots, dandelion greens, beef, fish, and cow liver. One of the best herbs for liver health is milk thistle, a member of the aster and daisy family, and was used by ancient physicians and herbalists to treat a range of liver and gallbladder diseases, as well as to protect the liver against a variety of poisons.

The National Library of Medicine reports, "Evidence exists that milk thistle may be hepatoprotective through a number of mechanisms: antioxidant activity, toxin blockade at the membrane level, enhanced protein synthesis, antifibriotic activity, and possible anti-inflammatory or immunomodulating effects."[273]

---

[273] National Library of Medicine, Milk Thistle: Effects on Liver Disease and Cirrhosis and Clinical Adverse Effects, Evidence Report/Technology Assessment Number 21, Prepared for: Agency for Healthcare Research and Quality, U.S. Department of Health and Human Services, 2101 East Jefferson Street, Rockville, MD 20852, Contract No. 290-97-0012; ncbi.nlm.nih.gov/books/bv.fcgi?rid=hstat1.chapter.29128, Prepared by:San Antonio Evidence-based Practice Center based at The University of Texas Health Science Center at San Antonio and The Veterans Evidence-based Research, Dissemination, and Implementation Center, a Veterans Affairs Health Services Research and Development Center of Excellence, Cynthia Mulrow, MD, MSc, Program Director

Who Said 'It's Not Easy Being Green'?

Too few people eat green foods, but this is where most of the nutrition is. Thus it's time to start preparing meals with spinach, broccoli, kale, bok choy, arugula, chard, and other foods wherein chlorophyll (the green pigment in vegetables) is king.

There has been so much research proving the benefits of green vegetables that you'd think we'd have a population of Popeyes running around. But we don't. Why not? Some doctors speculate that it's because green vegetables can taste a little bitter due to their potassium and mineral content. On the other hand, natural sugars, which are more abundant in fruits than they are in green vegetables, are far more popular. So if you were weaned on processed children's breakfast cereals, pizza, and burgers, you'll have to retrain your senses and acquire a taste for your greens. Or else!!

What do green vegetables have that we all need so badly? Minerals, trace minerals, chlorophyll, vitamins, antioxidants, carotenes, flavonoids, and fiber, to name a few ingredients.

Green Vegetable Highlights:
- Some of the phytochemicals in green vegetables can help in digestion and keep bad bacteria out of your stomach. Broccoli is a great source of these phytochemicals.
- Leafy greens (and some fruits) also contain a phytochemical that keeps your eyes healthy and may even keep you from going blind as you age. Spinach, kale, and collard greens are the best sources.
- Some green vegetables are high in beta-carotene, another important antioxidant that your body can convert to vitamin A, supporting your vision, your immunity, and the health of your skin.
- Several types of leafy, green vegetables are also good sources of calcium (essential for strong bones) and potassium (promotes regular heartbeat and muscle contraction and supports kidney function).

A study reported in the journal *Diabetes Care*, women who have a higher intake of green, leafy vegetables and fruit have a lower risk for type 2 diabetes, whereas those who have a higher intake of fruit juices may have an increased risk for the disease.[274]

Fruit and vegetable consumption has been associated with decreased incidence of deaths from a variety of health issues, including obesity, hypertension, and cardiovascular diseases in epidemiological studies.[275]

Diets high in red meat and low in green vegetables are associated with increased colon cancer risk.[276]

---

[274] Barclay, MD, Laurie, Green Leafy Vegetables, Fruit Intake Linked to Lower Risk for Diabetes in Women, *Medscape Medical News*, Jul 08

[275] ibid

[276] Johan de Vogel, Denise S.M.L. Jonker-Termont, Esther M.M. van Lieshout, Martijn B. Katan and Roelof van der Meer, Green vegetables, red meat and colon cancer: chlorophyll prevents the cytotoxic and hyperproliferative effects of haem in rat colon, Carcinogenesis 2005 26(2):387-393; doi:10.1093/carcin/bgh331; http://carcin.oxfordjournals.org/cgi/content/abstract/26/2/387

It's Your Turn to Super Charge Your Health

From all you've read in this book, you have a fairly good idea that nature offers a natural system of healing and disease prevention in its complex, complete Super Foods. This is a claim that cannot be made of scientifically created supplements that isolate some of a food's parts (like the vitamins, minerals, or amino acids) and leaves the other food ingredients on the laboratory floor, so to speak. ***Real foods come from real plants, not manufacturing plants.***

Now the question is: How do you take advantage of these Super Foods and incorporate them into your life to improve your health and the health of your family?

Certainly, you need conviction. You have to realize that over the past fifty years or so we've been going in the wrong direction, health-wise, as evidenced by the soaring rate of diseases owing to bad food, a polluted environment, stress, and a sedentary lifestyle. To reverse this disastrous course in your own life, you need to take the path less-traveled by eating Super Foods, drinking pure water, exercising, managing your stress, getting rid of body care products that are loaded with chemicals, putting a stop to eating bad fats and artificial ingredients, and paying attention to toxic threats from your environment.

Here Are Three Main Ways To Bring Super Foods Into Your Life:

1. Put them in your daily diet. This means finding the foods we've written about at your health food and grocery store and making recipes with them. For instance, make meals with carrots, broccoli, garlic, and Maitake mushrooms, instead of eating pizza. And, if you can't do without pizza, make it yourself organically and add Super Foods to the recipe.

2. Juice them. A high-quality juicer can be a great way to get your daily Super Foods. A great juice recipe, for example, consists of beets, celery, parsley, carrots, garlic, and grapes —all organic. Vegetables consumed as juices take a quick route into your blood stream and feed every cell in your entire body.

3. Take them in whole food–supplement form. You have to be aware of what's on a supplement product's label. If there are chemical names in the main ingredient panel (such as ascorbic acid, vitamin A palmitate, mixed tocopherols, pyrodixine, etc.) then you're not getting foods, but chemical isolates instead. We recommend NutriPlex Formulas because their products do not contain chemical isolates, artificial ingredients, genetically modified foods, or irradiated substances. Remember that Super Foods are valuable for their entire food complexes, not just for their vitamins, minerals or antioxidants.

The Super Foods Diet is not a short-term fad. Instead, it's a way of incorporating the most powerful healing and disease-preventive foods and herbs into your daily life, because scientific studies show that their ingredients fight and prevent cancer, heart disease, obesity, diabetes, arthritis, bacteria infections, and a host of the most problematic diseases of our time. Now that science has finally begun to discover the Super Foods that have been used since ancient times, it's time to build your health around them!

Appendix

Antibiotic Super Foods
Additional Sources:
1. M. Kumar & J.S. Berwal; Department of Animal Products Technology, CCS Haryana Agricultural University, Hisar, IndiaPublished Online: 5 Jan 2002
2. *J. Agric. Food Chem.*, 1999, 47 (10), pp 4297–4300

Apples Fight Cancer
Additional Sources:
1. USDA Nutrient Data Laboratory – Apple
2. University of Illinois Extension, University of Illinois at Urbana-Champaign
3. Bladder Cancer Web Café 2004

Iron-Clad Food Builds Blood
Additional Sources:
1. Trumbo P, Yates AA, Schlicker S, Poos M. Food and Nutrition Board, Institute of Medicine, The National Academies, Washington, DC. Dietary reference intakes: vitamin A, vitamin K, arsenic, boron, chromium, copper, iodine, iron, manganese, molybdenum, nickel, silicon, vanadium, and zinc. J Am Diet Assoc. 2001 Mar;101(3):294-301.
2. Allen RE, Myers AL. Nutrition in toddlers. Am Fam Physician. 2006 Nov 1;74(9):1527-32. Review.
3. U.S. National Library of Medicine, National Institutes of Health; Jan 07
4. Campos Outcalt, Douglas, Twenty Problems in Preventive Health Care, McGraw Hill, 2000

Pain Relief With Foods
Additional sources:

1. Science Daily; American Chemical Society, Feb. 1999
2. Janet Raloff, *Science News*; sciencenews.org

Borage Oil for Eczema?

Additional Sources:

1. American Academy of Dermatology (1995).
2. Morse, P.F., et al. Meta-analysis of placebo-controlled studies of the efficacy of Epogam in the treatment of atopic eczema. Relationship between plasma essential fatty acid changes and clinical response, British
3. *Journal of Dermatology*, Vol. 121, pp. 75-90 (1989).
4. Andreassi, M., et al. Efficacy of Gamma Linolenic Acid in the Treatment of Patients with Atopic Dermatitis,
5. *Journal of International Medical Research*, Vol. 25, pp. 266-74 (1997).
6. Henz, B.M., Double-blind, multicentre analysis of the efficacy of borage oil in patients with atopic eczema, Br J Dermatol. 1999 Apr;140(4):685-8

Feeding Your Liver

Additional sources:

1. Worman, MD, Howard, New York Presbyterian Hospital, 2005, abcnews.com
2. Duke University Health Center, 2005
3. hepatitis.org.uk
4. National Institutes of Health, Agency for Healthcare Research and Quality, Evidence Report/Technology Assessment: Number 21, "Milk Thistle: Effects on Liver Disease and Cirrhosis and Clinical Adverse Effects"
5. American Liver Foundation: liverfoundation.org

Who Said It's Not Easy Being Green?

Additional Sources:

1. VIC Kids Program, Vegetable & Fruit Improvement Center, Texas A&M University System, 2000

About the Author

Vic Shayne, PhD, has written numerous books and hundreds of articles on nutrition and natural health care. For more than two decades he has served as a clinician, doctor's consultant, whole food supplement formulator (for NutriPlex Formulas, Inc.) and health writer. Some of his books include *Man Cannot Live on Vitamins Alone, Whole Nutrition: The Missing Link in Vitamin Therapy, Evil Genius in the Garden of Eden,* and *Illness Isn't Caused by a Drug Deficiency!*

Made in the USA
Columbia, SC
05 November 2022

70491884R00114